T0251647

Prevention Issues for Women's Health in the New Millennium

Prevention Issues for Women's Health in the New Millennium has been co-published simultaneously as *Journal of Prevention & Intervention in the Community*, Volume 22, Number 2 2001.

Prevention Issues for Women's Health in the New Millennium

Wendee M. Wechsberg
Editor

Prevention Issues for Women's Health in the New Millennium has been co-published simultaneously as *Journal of Prevention & Intervention in the Community*, Volume 22, Number 2 2001.

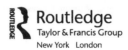

Routledge
Taylor & Francis Group
New York London

First published by
The Haworth Press, Inc., 10 Alice Street, Binghamton, NY 13904-1580

This edition published 2013 by Routledge
711 Third Avenue, New York, NY 10017
2 Park Square, Milton Park, Abingdon, Oxon OX14 4RN

Routledge is an imprint of the Taylor & Francis Group, an informa business

Prevention Issues for Women's Health in the New Millennium has been co-published simultaneously as *Journal of Prevention & Intervention in the Community*™, Volume 22, Number 2 2001.

© 2001 by The Haworth Press, Inc. All rights reserved. No part of this work may be reproduced or utilized in any form or by any means, electronic or mechanical, including photocopying, microfilm and recording, or by any information storage and retrieval system, without permission in writing from the publisher.

The development, preparation, and publication of this work has been undertaken with great care. However, the publisher, employees, editors, and agents of The Haworth Press and all imprints of The Haworth Press, Inc., including The Haworth Medical Press® and Pharmaceutical Products Press®, are not responsible for any errors contained herein or for consequences that may ensue from use of materials or information contained in this work. Opinions expressed by the author(s) are not necessarily those of The Haworth Press, Inc.

Cover design by Thomas J. Mayshock Jr.

Library of Congress Cataloging-in-Publication Data

Prevention issues for women's health in the new millennium / Wendee M. Wechsberg.
    p. cm.
    "Co-published simultaneously as Journal of prevention & intervention in the community, Volume 22, Number 2, 2001."
    Includes bibliographical references and index.
    ISBN 0-7890-1382-7 (alk. paper)–ISBN 0-7890-1383-5 (alk. paper)
    1. Women–Health and Hygiene. 2. Women–Diseases–Prevention. I. Wechsberg, Wendee M.

RA778.P8856 2001
613'.04244–dc21
                                          2001039921

Prevention Issues for Women's Health in the New Millennium

CONTENTS

ABOUT THE EDITOR

Wendee M. Wechsberg, PhD, is currently program director of the Substance Abuse Treatment Research group and senior research psychologist at Research Triangle Institute and the principal investigator of five projects. Her life story and clinical experience–as director of treatment services of both outpatient and residential drug treatment programs for adolescents and adults–have afforded her a real-world sense of the needs of women. Her research efforts have centered on developing strategies for contacting hard-to-reach populations, particularly out-of-treatment women and minorities, and on developing appropriate interventions for them. She has published on substance abusers and HIV risk, outreach effectiveness, gender differences, and women's issues. As an applied researcher, she is hoping research will help change practice, particularly with sensitivity for gender, culture, and class.

Introduction:
Prevention Issues for Women's Health
in the New Millennium

Wendee M. Wechsberg

Research Triangle Institute

Over the past 10 years, women's health issues have become a national priority. There has been a growing acceptance that women's health does not mean solely a woman's reproductive health but rather the numerous health issues and needs that are distinctly different from men's. Women's health encompasses the woman's unique biology as well as her sociocultural, economic, and physical environments (NWHIC, 2000). These individual and contextual factors affect not only the duration of but also the quality of a woman's life.

In response to growing congressional and public concerns over perceived inattention to women's health issues, the Public Health Service (PHS) announced in 1991 an Action Plan for Women's Health. The plan designated broad areas of concern in women's health but also emphasized that women's health needs vary and that special minority populations may be particularly vulnerable. For example, the average

---

Address correspondence to: Wendee M. Wechsberg, PhD, Program Director, Substance Abuse Treatment Research, Health and Social Policy Division, Research Triangle Institute, Research Triangle Park, NC 27709-2194.

This special volume was supported by a Professional Development Award at Research Triangle Institute (W0300). There are several people who need to be thanked in addition to the authors: William Zule, Dr. Ph., Erika Fulmer, Merry Wood, Ashley Simons, and, most importantly, my editor Sallie West.

[Haworth co-indexing entry note]: "Introduction: Prevention Issues for Women's Health in the New Millennium." Wechsberg, Wendee M. Co-published simultaneously in *Journal of Prevention & Intervention in the Community* (The Haworth Press, Inc.) Vol. 22, No. 2, 2001, pp. 1-5; and: *Prevention Issues for Women's Health in the New Millennium* (ed: Wendee M. Wechsberg) The Haworth Press, Inc., 2001, pp. 1-5. Single or multiple copies of this article are available for a fee from The Haworth Document Delivery Service [1-800-342-9678, 9:00 a.m. - 5:00 p.m. (EST). E-mail address: getinfo@haworthpressinc.com].

© 2001 by The Haworth Press, Inc. All rights reserved.

1

life expectancy of a woman varies considerably, depending on her race: in 1997, the average life expectancy for Caucasian women was five years longer than that of African-American women (80 versus 75 years). Women who live in poverty or have less than a high school education have shorter life spans; higher rates of illness, injury, disability, and death; and more limited access to high-quality health-care services (Lyons, Salganicoff, & Rowland, 1996).

The result has been an increase in programs and funding for examining "diseases or conditions unique to women, more prevalent in women, more serious among women, or having different risk factors or interventions on women" (DHHS, 1991). In addition, there has been an expanding reclassification of issues that historically were considered to be social problems (e.g., aging, rural, poverty, sexual orientation, minority, substance abuse) but now are seen as public health issues that affect women disproportionately.

To address this burgeoning field of study, the *Journal of Prevention & Intervention in the Community* announced a call for papers to highlight contributions in health-related prevention and intervention research on women. The goal was to highlight important research in areas identified as having particular relevance among women and those having lasting implications. The six articles included in this volume share the common theme of disease prevention in women, and different ethnic and disease groups are represented. Some are pilot studies, introducing data where there is a void–for example, among harder-to-reach at-risk women. These studies indicate a need for greater outreach among–and understanding the health issues of–certain populations.

The first two articles deal with cancer, a leading cause of death in women in the United States. Prevention and early detection are the first important steps to reducing deaths from cancer. Breast cancer, which strikes one in eight women, is second only to lung cancer in deaths among women and third to heart disease. In "Performance of Breast Self-Exam: An Interaction with Age," A. Bryan compares the role of perceived susceptibility to breast cancer to the practice of breast self-exam in older women. Differences were found with regard to age and how women perceive their risk, and they highlight the importance of using psychological research on the correlates and predictors of health risk and protective behaviors.

R. Michielutte, L. Cunningham, P. Sharp, M. Dignan, and V. Burnette look at the effectiveness of education and support services of rural health departments in increasing early cancer-detection behaviors in "Effectiveness of a Cancer Education Program for Women Attending Rural Public Health Departments in North Carolina." The results may have some profound implications in terms of a more personalized education but also for reaching rural women using a combination of readable printed materials and telephone contact for early detection of breast and skin cancer. Telephone counseling is not only inexpensive but a way to reach underserved populations. The wave of the future may include utilizing technology to reach less accessible populations, and, until computers are in every home, telephones can be an avenue for health prevention efforts in rural communities.

D. Powers, D. Bowen, and J. White compare health-related behavior and sexual orientation in "The Influence of Sexual Orientation on Health Behaviors in Women." Here, they raise the question of whether lesbians are at risk for poorer health outcomes than are heterosexual women because of differential health behaviors and risk factors for disease. Lesbians were found to participate in mammography and Pap testing at significantly lower levels than bisexuals and heterosexuals. Although this study was preliminary, it did support the idea that additional research into health behavior differences between lesbians and non-lesbians is essential.

"Reduction of Co-Occurring Distress and HIV Risk Behaviors Among Women Substance Abusers," by S. Reif, W. Wechsberg, and M. Dennis, evaluates the influence of one's participation in a risk-reduction project for reducing co-occurring distress issues. This study not only reinforces the need for individual assessment plans with high-risk inner city minority women, it demonstrates that women who report higher co-morbidity symptoms related to mental health respond better to more comprehensive and longer interventions, even with regard to risk behaviors.

C. Waters, R. Times, A. R. Morton, M. Crear, and M. Wey look at the association between perceived health status and health promotion practices in a minority sample in "Perception of Health Status and Participation in Present and Future Health Promotion Behaviors Among African-American Women." Reviewing data from a cross-sectional, descriptive survey, the authors suggest that women are interested in participating in future health-promotion activities for African-American women. Yet, to expect change, those involved with the intervention must understand not only the woman's individual behavioral and health risks but also understand it within the context of the expectations of their culture.

Finally, S. Stevens assesses the health-care needs and service provisions for American-Indian women who are substance abusers in "American-Indian Women and Health." She stresses that little is known about health status and health-related issues of urban American-Indian women. Numerous health-care issues–including heavy substance abuse, sexual-risk and reproductive-health problems–suggest the need for comprehensive, culturally competent, and gender-specific prevention and treatment services.

While this special volume cannot address the entire range of complex issues emerging in the arena of women's health, it offers promising directions and avenues geared toward prevention health issues. It further implies ways to reach women who may have less opportunity to be part of the mainstream medical care environment by stressing the need for preventive medicine.

Current research has shown that 50 percent of the leading diseases causing death in women–including heart disease, cancer, stroke, and lung disease–are related to behavior (NWHIC, 2000). Empowering women to make more informed health decisions about their health through all stages of life is paramount. Therefore, prevention efforts emphasizing healthy behaviors during the formative years can be crucial. Tradition shows, as women grow, they will take on many more external challenges because they have also historically been the primary health-care providers and health decision-makers for their families. Yet, they have not necessarily been the greatest caretakers of themselves. Furthermore, with the life expectancy of women in the U.S. having increased from 48.3 years in 1900 to 79.4 years in 1997 (Centers for Disease Control and Prevention, 1999), women are also caring for elderly parents, in addition to their own children (Family Care Giver Alliance, 1999). With increasing stresses of home, vocation, and extended commitments, women are challenged now, more than ever, to maintain their own health by making those extra years of life healthy and productive with proven prevention strategies. Reaching minority and low-income women in their communities remains a challenge, where barriers of ethnicity, acculturation, language, and access are obstacles. Because of a diminishing access to health-care services, these women need to be equipped with knowledge to keep them healthy as they confront their daily struggles. Personal prevention health is knowledge and knowledge is power, which will hopefully translate to improve not only a woman's individual life but also that of her family and future generations. Studies such as these within the communities of women with greater risk are just beginning, and further analysis in the new millennium will be needed to address issues that may hopefully become prevention practice.

REFERENCES

CDC (1999). *Health, United States, 1999 with health and aging chartbook*. Hyattsville, MD: Center for Health Statistics.

Department of Health and Human Services (1991). (Publication No. 91-50414).

Family Care Giver Alliance (1999). *Selected care giver statistics*. Fact Sheet. October.

Lyons, B., Salganicoff, A., & Rowland, D. (1996). Poverty, access to health care, and Medicaid's critical role for women. In M.M. Falik & K.S. Collins (Eds.), *Women's health*: *The commonwealth fund survey*. Baltimore, MD: Johns Hopkins University Press.

National Women's Health Information Center, Office on Women's Health, Department of Health and Human Services Web Page: http://www.4women.gov/media/statinfo.htm.

Performance of Breast Self-Exam:
An Interaction with Age

Angela D. Bryan

University of Colorado

SUMMARY. Breast cancer is a significant health threat for women and is currently the second-leading cause of cancer-related deaths in women. When breast cancer is diagnosed early in the disease process, the probability of survival is quite high, but when diagnosis is made at a later stage, mortality increases dramatically. Thus, early detection is crucial, and monthly breast self-exam (BSE) is recommended for all women over the age of 20. Despite this recommendation, adherence to BSE guidelines is quite low. The current study investigated the role of perceived susceptibility to breast cancer as it relates to the performance of BSE among a sample of community women. As hypothesized, a significant interaction between perceived susceptibility and age was found such that perceived susceptibility was significantly positively related to BSE performance for older women but was not related to BSE performance among younger women. Although there are certainly other variables associated with BSE performance, the implications of this particular finding for the design of interventions to increase BSE performance are discussed. *[Article copies available for a fee from The Haworth Document Delivery Service: 1-800-342-9678. E-mail address: <getinfo@haworthpress inc.*

Angela D. Bryan, PhD, is affiliated with the Department of Psychology/Institute of Behavioral Science, University of Colorado.

Address correspondence to: Angela D. Bryan, PhD, University of Colorado, Department of Psychology/Institute of Behavioral Science, CB345, Boulder, CO 80309-0345.

This research was supported by a grant from the National Institute of Mental Health (MH 46244-05).

[Haworth co-indexing entry note]: "Performance of Breast Self-Exam: An Interaction with Age." Bryan, Angela D. Co-published simultaneously in *Journal of Prevention & Intervention in the Community* (The Haworth Press, Inc.) Vol. 22, No. 2, 2001, pp. 7-22; and: *Prevention Issues for Women's Health in the New Millennium* (ed: Wendee M. Wechsberg) The Haworth Press, Inc., 2001, pp. 7-22. Single or multiple copies of this article are available for a fee from The Haworth Document Delivery Service [1-800-342-9678, 9:00 a.m. - 5:00 p.m. (EST). E-mail address: getinfo@haworthpressinc.com].

© 2001 by The Haworth Press, Inc. All rights reserved.

com> Website: <http://www.HaworthPress.com> © 2001 by The Haworth Press, Inc. All rights reserved.]

KEYWORDS. Breast cancer, breast self-exam, perceived susceptibility, interaction effect

In 1998 the American Cancer Society (ACS) estimated that close to 180,000 new cases of invasive breast cancer would be diagnosed that year (ACS, 1998). Breast cancer is currently the second-leading cause of women's cancer-related deaths (ACS, 1998). It is the leading cause of cancer-related death in women aged 40-55, and approximately one in eight women will incur breast cancer at some point in their lives. When breast cancer is diagnosed and treated while the cancer is still localized, women have an over 90% five-year survival rate. When detection and treatment come at later stages of the disease, the survival rate is much lower (ACS, 1998).

These statistics clearly point out the importance of early detection in the treatment of breast cancer and screening for breast cancer, either by mammography, clinical breast exam, or breast self-examination (BSE). There are three primary guidelines for early breast cancer detection recommended by the ACS (1998). First, all women, after the age of 20, should perform monthly breast self-exams. Second, breast examinations by a medical professional are recommended every three years for women between 20 and 40, and every year for women over 40. Finally, women are encouraged to have a mammogram every year beginning at age 40.

Although mammography is the most effective technique for detecting early breast cancer (Benedict, Williams, & Hoomani, 1996; Perdue, Galbo, & Ghosh, 1995; Senie, Lesser, Kinne, & Rosen, 1994), BSE is also a crucial mode of detection. Breast lumps are often first detected by women or their sexual partners through either BSE or accidental palpation (e.g., Benedict et al., 1996; Reeves, Newcomb, Remington, & Marcus, 1996). BSE is thus an important detection method recommended by oncologists, as neither clinical breast exams nor mammography is universally successful at breast cancer detection (Benedict et al., 1996). In addition, as a result of economic or other barriers, clinical breast exams and mammography may not be readily available to all women (ACS, 1998; Pinto & Fuqua, 1991).

Despite the benefits of BSE as a method of breast cancer detection, the actual BSE performance rate is quite low among community samples of women in the United States (e.g., Cope, 1992; Friedman, Nelson, Webb, Hoffman, & Baer, 1994; Hailey & Bradford, 1991; Salazar et al., 1994). For instance, Salazar et al. (1994) found that fewer than one-third of their study's participants regularly performed BSE. Hailey and Bradford (1991) reported similar results. Research in which participants were recruited in medical settings, however, has occasionally found higher BSE performance rates. For example, Duke, Gordon-Sosby, Reynolds, and Gram (1994) found that 66% of 33 African-American women surveyed at a public health clinic performed regular BSE. Though rates of performance vary somewhat, it is clear that a substantial portion of U.S. women do not regularly engage in BSE.

PSYCHOLOGICAL CORRELATES OF BSE PERFORMANCE

The Health Belief Model (HBM) (Janz & Becker, 1984) is a behavioral change framework that has been used to predict BSE frequency. Within that framework, barriers (i.e., forgetting, depending on clinical exams, lack of confidence in BSE ability) have been found to be the factor most commonly associated with not practicing BSE (e.g., Clarke, Hill, Rassaby, White, & Hirst, 1991; Roche & Gosnell, 1989; Strauss, Solomon, Costanza, Worden, & Foster, 1987). For example, Shepperd, Solomon, Atkins, Foster, and Frankowski (1990) reported that perceived barriers accounted for 67% of the variance in BSE frequency.

While the identification of perceived barriers as a strong predictor of BSE frequency is an important finding, other HBM constructs have not consistently accounted for variation in BSE practice (Aiken, Fenaughty, West, Johnson, & Luckett, 1995; Lierman, Young, Kasprzyk, & Benoliel, 1990). Perceived severity (i.e., the degree to which breast cancer is perceived as a severe health threat) has *not* been a successful predictor of monthly BSE practice (Ronis & Kaiser, 1989; Stillman, 1977), and perceived susceptibility (i.e., the likelihood that one will incur breast cancer) has been an inconsistent predictor of BSE, having produced some positive results (Agars & McMurray, 1993; Champion & Menon, 1997) and some null results (Amsel, Grover, & Balshem, 1985; Lu, 1995; Ruda, Bourcier, & Skiff, 1992). As with many health behaviors, the relationship between perceived susceptibility to a negative outcome (breast cancer) and the practice of a health protective behavior (BSE) appears to be complicated (Fisher & Fisher, in press; Gerrard, Gibbons, & Bushman, 1996; Weinstein & Nicolich, 1993) and not well-understood.

Preventive interventions promoting BSE by influencing psychological variables virtually always include information about susceptibility to breast cancer in an effort to encourage women to acknowledge their personal vulnerability to breast cancer (e.g., Rassaby, Hirst, Hill, Bennett, & Clarke, 1991; Siero, Kok, & Pruyn, 1984). Increased perceptions of susceptibility to breast cancer are then expected to be translated into increased BSE performance. In the service of designing the most effective interventions possible to promote this vital health behavior, it is important to understand whether or not a perception of susceptibility is related to BSE performance, or if there are certain populations for whom it is especially important. It may be that for specific populations intervention time might be better spent targeting specific barriers to BSE.

Age and Breast Cancer Susceptibility

An individual woman's susceptibility to breast cancer is influenced by a number of factors, including family history (Brody & Biesecker, 1998; Salazar et al., 1994) and diet (Maskarinec, Singh, Meng, & Franke, 1998; Mezzetti et al., 1998). However, the most consistent factor associated with breast cancer susceptibility is a woman's age, with increasing age relating to increased susceptibility to breast cancer (ACS, 1998; Clarke et al., 1991; Costanza, 1994; Lierman et al., 1990). Thus, actual susceptibility to breast cancer changes across the lifespan, and if this change in susceptibility is accurately perceived, it may be that the relationship between susceptibility and BSE may also change across the lifespan. Specifically, perceived susceptibility might become a more salient factor for older women, and thus might be more strongly related to BSE practice among older women. There has been some research investigating this possible role of age on the effect of perceived susceptibility on BSE performance.

A number of researchers have found a positive relationship between perceived susceptibility and BSE among *older* women (Agars & McMurray 1993; Champion & Menon, 1997; Champion & Miller, 1992; Fletcher, Morgan, O'Malley, Earp, & Degnan, 1989; Massey, 1986; Roche & Gosnell, 1989). On the other hand, researchers have found no relationship between perceived susceptibility and BSE among *young* women, generally in samples of college women (Mamon & Zapka, 1986; Ronis & Kaiser, 1989; Ruda et al., 1992). Champion and Miller (1992) sought to examine the association of health beliefs to BSE among women in three age groups (35-44, 45-54, and 55+). In contrast to the hypothesis posed above, Champion and Miller (1992) found that the relationship between perceived susceptibility to breast cancer and performance of BSE was dependent upon age, such that there was a positive relationship between perceived susceptibility and BSE for the younger age group but not for the older groups. Very young women (i.e., those under 35) were not included in the sample, so from Champion and Miller's (1992) data it is not clear what the role of susceptibility would be for women under 35. Overall, there appears to be some empirical support for a relationship between susceptibility and BSE for older women but not for younger women, suggesting the presence of a possible interactive effect.

Detection of Interactive Effects in Field Studies

There is a long history of research (Zedeck, 1971; Champoux & Peters, 1987; Jaccard, Turrisi, & Wan, 1990) highlighting the difficulty of detecting interactions in field studies. Fairly recently, McClelland and Judd (1993) provided an extensive and thorough review of this issue. Briefly, McClelland and Judd (1993) showed through theoretical derivation and computer simulations that the properties of the joint distribution between a moderator and an independent variable in a field study diverge quite substantially from the optimal design for detecting interaction effects. An optimal design is one that provides maximum statistical power and minimal standard errors, generally one that most closely resembles a 2×2, equal *n* factorial design common in experimental laboratory research. The main consequence of these findings for the present research is that a test for an interaction between susceptibility and age in a community sample of women must be undertaken with an understanding of the difficulties inherent in detecting such effects. One crucial factor is that continuous variables *should not* be separated into an artificially small number of categories. Such cut-pointing of continuous variables introduces increased measurement error (Aiken & West, 1991; Busemeyer & Jones, 1983), which increases standard errors and makes already difficult to detect interactions even harder to find (McClelland & Judd, 1993). Thus, in the current study, the moderator variable of age will be retained as a continuous variable, in order to afford the best chance of detecting the hypothesized interactive effect.

The goal of this study was to conduct a methodologically rigorous test for the presence of a perceived susceptibility to breast cancer by age interaction on the performance of BSE. Since women's suscepti-bility to breast cancer does in fact increase as a function of increasing age, it was predicted that, for older women, perceptions of susceptibil-ity would be more salient. Thus, perceived susceptibility might be more strongly related to the performance of BSE. For younger women, no such relationship was predicted. To be sure, age and perceived suscepti-bility to breast cancer are not the only important psychosocial or demo-graphic determinants of BSE. These were the only variables addressed in the current work for both theoretical/methodological and practical reasons. From a theoretical perspective, the goal of the study was to detect an interactive effect. Methodologically, this necessitated that the number of predictors in the regression equations be limited in order to optimize the ratio of subjects to parameters estimated and thus the power to detect a significant interaction if one were present. From a practical perspective, hypotheses regarding the influence of other important psychosocial predictors, such as breast cancer information, attitudes about BSE, social norms supporting the practice of BSE, and self-efficacy for BSE have already been addressed in this particular sample (cf. Misovich, Fisher, Martinez, Bryan, & Catapano, in re-view).

METHOD

Participants. Female employees (n = 200) of the University of Connecticut were mailed a 16-page survey labeled the "Health Main-tenance Behavior Inventory." Of the women who were mailed the survey, 166 completed and returned it as instructed, for a response rate of 83%. Average age of respondents was 42.6, with a range from 22 to 64. The majority of the participants (94%) were Caucasian, 3% were African-American, and 2% were Latina. One respondent reported be-ing Native American, one reported being Asian or a Pacific Islander, and one listed "other." Overall, 25% of the women had had an imme-diate family member who had been diagnosed with breast cancer, and

56% had a close friend (not a family member) who had been diagnosed with breast cancer.

Procedure. Each participant was mailed a copy of the questionnaire,
along with a cover letter describing the purpose of the research, and an
envelope in which the questionnaire could be returned through the
on-campus mail system. Participants were instructed to complete the
questionnaire anonymously and to return it within the next two weeks.
As an incentive to complete the questionnaire, participants were also
given the opportunity to enter a raffle, with the winners receiving gift
certificates for a local department store. A separate card was provided
which served as a raffle ticket, and the participants were asked to write
their name on the card and return it separately to the researchers. A
reminder letter was sent to participants approximately six weeks after
the initial questionnaire was distributed.

Measures. A complete description of all the measures in the questionnaire appears in Misovich et al. (in review). For the purposes of
the current study, only the measures of perceived susceptibility to
breast cancer and performance of BSE were evaluated.

Perceived susceptibility. Participants were asked: "Considering all
the factors that may contribute to developing breast cancer, what
would you say are your chances of getting breast cancer?" The response options for this item were: 1 = "almost certainly will not," 2 =
"small or very small chance," 3 = "some chance," 4 = "large or very
large chance," and 5 = "almost certainly will."

Performance of BSE. Women were asked: "How frequently have
you self-examined your breasts during the past six months?" Response options were: 1 = "have not at all," 2 = "between 1 and 2
times," 3 = "between 3 and 5 times," 4 = "monthly." Thus, higher
numbers corresponded to more frequent BSE.

RESULTS

BSE Behavior

Only a minority of respondents were practicing BSE at the recommended monthly interval. Twenty-two percent of the respondents indicated that they performed BSE at least once a month over the last six
months, while 32% examined their breasts somewhat less frequently

(i.e., between three and five times during the last six months). Nearly a third (32%) had practiced BSE only once or twice during the previous six months, and 14% had not examined their breasts at all during this interval. In Table 1, the mean age, education level, and percentage of participants who had a family member or friend diagnosed with breast cancer are presented for each category of BSE practice. Note that there were no significant differences in the practice of BSE for any of these variables.

Perceived Susceptibility to Breast Cancer

The mean score on the five-point scale ranging from "almost certainly will not get breast cancer" to "almost certainly will get breast cancer" was 2.82 (sd = .67). This mean score indicates that, overall, the women in this sample feel that there is "some chance" that they will get breast cancer. There was a significant positive correlation between perceived susceptibility and actual breast self-examination behavior in the past six months (r (161) = .23, p < .01). To test the hypothesis that the relationship between perceived susceptibility and

TABLE 1. Practice of BSE by Mean Age, Education Level, and Presence of Family History or Close Friend's History of Breast Cancer

| | Performance of BSE in the Past Six Months | | | | Test for Difference |
	Not at all (n = 23)	1 to 2 times (n = 52)	3 to 5 times (n = 52)	Monthly (n = 36)	
Age[a]	42.40	43.12	40.30	44.03	F(3,159) <1, ns
	(10.36)	(8.03)	(11.13)	(9.09)	
Education Level					χ^2(12) = 7.23, ns
< High School	0%	0%	0%	0%	
High School	39%	21%	21%	22%	
Some College	9%	23%	15%	20%	
College Degree	13%	8%	10%	14%	
Some Graduate School	13%	10%	12%	8%	
Graduate Degree	26%	38%	42%	36%	
Family History of					
Breast Cancer	18%	17%	34%	25%	χ^2(3) = 4.39, ns
Close Friend with					
Breast Cancer	64%	47%	61%	56%	χ^2(3) = 2.64, ns

[a]Standard deviations appear in parentheses.

BSE varied as a function of age, a two-stage ordinary least squares (OLS) regression analysis was conducted. As per Aiken and West (1991), the categorical predictors of perceived susceptibility and age were centered (i.e., the mean was subtracted from each score, so that the mean of each construct was zero) before combining them to form the interaction term. Thus, the parameter estimates in the OLS regression equation described below refer to the test of the effect of perceived susceptibility on BSE at the mean value of age. The centered predictors were also used in calculating the main effects of these variables on BSE. All references to age and perceived susceptibility in this section will be to the centered versions of these variables.

In the first block of the regression equation, age and perceived susceptibility were entered to examine the main effects and variance accounted for. Unstandardized parameter estimates, standard errors, and standardized parameter estimates appear in Table 2. Perceived susceptibility exhibited a significant positive relationship with BSE, such that women who perceived a higher subjective personal susceptibility to breast cancer were more likely to have practiced BSE. The main effects model accounted for 7% of the variance in BSE. In the second block, the interaction term was entered into the equation and was a significant predictor of BSE above and beyond the main effects. There was also a significant change in variance accounted for, $R^2_\Delta =$ .03, $F(1,157) = 5.42$, $p < .05$, for a total of 10% of variance accounted for in BSE by the full set of predictors. This result is a small to medium effect size for multivariate models in the social sciences (Cohen, 1988).

This final regression equation with centered predictors gives the effect of perceived susceptibility on BSE at the mean age of the sample (42.8 years, see Figure 1). To probe the interaction between age and perceived susceptibility and for purposes of graphing the interaction, two additional regression equations were calculated. The first tested for the effect of perceived susceptibility on BSE for women one standard deviation above the mean age (52.4 years), and the second tested for the effect of perceived susceptibility on BSE for women one standard deviation below the mean age (33.3 years). These tests resulted in significance tests for the regression coefficient of the effects of perceived susceptibility at each of these ages (cf. Aiken & West, 1991, pp. 54-58). As can be seen in Figure 1, we found that, as predicted, for the older women in our sample there was a strong

TABLE 2. Ordinary Least Squares (OLS) Regressions Predicting BSE ($n = 161$)

	B	SE	β	p	R^2	$R^2\Delta$	Significance of $R^2\Delta$	Final Model p-value
				Frequency of BSE in Past Six Months				
Predictors								
Block One					.07	.07	$p < .01$	
Age X	.01	.01	.11	ns				ns
Perceived Susceptibility[a]	.35	.12	.23	$p < .01$				$p < .05$
Block Two								
Age X Perceived Susceptibility	.03	.01	.18	$p < .05$	.10	.03	$p < .05$	$p < .05$

[a]Age and Perceived Susceptibility refer to the centered values of these predictors, i.e., the mean has been subtracted from each score so that the mean of the variable is zero.

Note. B = unstandardized parameter estimate, SE = standard error, β = standardized parameter estimate.

significant positive relationship between perceived susceptibility and BSE ($B = .53$, $p < .001$). The relationship at the mean age was less positive (from original equation, $B = .19$, $p < .05$) while there was virtually no relationship between perceived susceptibility and BSE for the younger women in our sample ($B = .004$, *ns*).

DISCUSSION

In a community sample of women, a hypothesized significant interaction between perceived susceptibility and age on BSE performance was found. For older women, a perception of susceptibility to breast cancer was significantly related to the frequency with which BSE was performed. This relationship did not exist for younger women. This pattern of findings could very well be due to a correctly perceived increasing level of susceptibility to breast cancer associated with increasing age (ACS, 1998; Costanza, 1994). Perhaps as women age, they begin to focus more on their susceptibility to breast cancer, and this increased realization that breast cancer is a real threat to their health compels them to perform BSE more regularly. For younger women, it may be that other factors besides a perception of susceptibility to breast cancer, such as social normative support for BSE or self-efficacy for BSE, are responsible for BSE performance.

Implications for Intervention

In the introduction, it was suggested that perhaps intervention time spent focussing on perceived susceptibility might be better spent ad-

FIGURE 1. Plot of the significant interaction between perceived susceptibility to breast cancer and age on the probability of engaging in breast self-exam. Regression lines are plotted for participants at the mean age of the sample (42.8 years), one standard deviation above the mean (52.4 years), and one standard deviation below the mean (33.3 years). Perceived susceptibility ranges from 2 standard deviations below the mean (1.48) to 2 standard deviations above the mean (4.16) on the 1-5 scale.

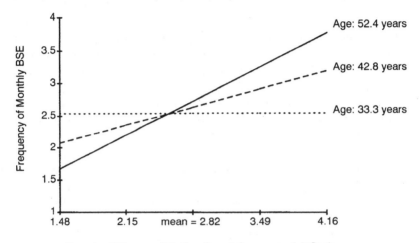

Perceived Chance of Getting Breast Cancer on 1-5 Scale

dressing more consistent psychological predictors of BSE, such as barriers. The findings of the current study indicate that what might be most efficacious is a focus on different psychological factors depending upon the audience (Champion & Miller, 1992). In an intervention with older women, it would appear that a focus on the increasing perceived susceptibility to breast cancer as a result of increasing age could lead intervention participants to increase their performance of BSE. For younger women, on the other hand, a focus on issues such as perceived barriers would make more sense. It is increasingly clear that the characteristics of the population with whom one intends to conduct a health promotion intervention be taken into account when designing the intervention. This has been true in intervention research with other health behaviors, including HIV risk reduction (Bryan, Aiken, & West, 1997; Fisher & Fisher, 1992; McCoy, McCoy, & Lai, 1998), substance abuse prevention (Baldwin et al., 1996), smoking cessation (Dijkstra, DeVries, Roijackers, & vanBreukelen, 1998; King, T., Bor-relli, Black, Pinto, & Marcus, 1997; Lichtenstein, 1997), mammography (King, E. et al., 1998), and hypertension control (Fouad et al., 1997). It is thus not surprising that tailoring intervention content to the population with which one is intervening might be important for BSE as well.

Limitations

This study was a cross-sectional study of a predominantly white, highly educated sample of women, and thus conclusions based on these data are preliminary. The findings should be replicated in further studies involving larger, more diverse samples, and utilizing longitudinal designs to clarify direction of effects. Further, in order to specifically focus on the testing of the hypothesized interaction effect, the only psychological variable included in the analysis was perceived susceptibility. Other work has demonstrated the importance of a number of psychological variables (Champion, 1990; Misovich et al., 1999; Ronis & Kaiser, 1989), and the current findings are not meant to suggest that perceived susceptibility is the only important psychological predictor of BSE. The current study was somewhat limited by sample size, and the limited power of the design to detect the hypothesized effect in the presence of other, arguably important, predictors. To test the simultaneous effects of other psychosocial and demographic predictors of BSE, larger samples that allow for more sophisticated multivariate techniques are needed.

CONCLUSION

The current study showed that the influence of perceived susceptibility to breast cancer on the performance of BSE may vary with age. More generally, the findings highlight the importance of conducting basic psychological research on the correlates and predictors of health risk and protective behavior. Such basic research reveals specific patterns of relationships for specific subgroups of populations at risk for disease and allows for the development of targeted intervention efforts.

REFERENCES

ACS. (1998). *The Breast Cancer Resource Center.* Available on the Web at http://www3.cancer.org/cancerinfo/res_home.asp?ct=5.
Agars, J., & McMurray, A. (1993). An evaluation of comparative strategies for teaching breast self-examination. *Journal of Advanced Nursing, 18*, 595-1603.

Aiken, L.S., Fenaughty, A.M., West, S.G., Johnson, J.J., & Luckett, T.L. (1995). Perceived determinants of risk for breast cancer and the relations among objective risk, perceived risk, and screening behavior over time. *Women's Health: Research on Gender, Behavior, and Policy, 1*, 27-50.

Aiken, L.S., & West, S.G. (1991). *Multiple regression: Testing and interpreting interactions*. Newbury Park: Sage.

Amsel, Z., Grover, P.L., & Balshem, A.M. (1985). Frequency of breast self examination practice as a function of physician reinforcement. *Patient Education and Counseling, 7*, 147-155.

Baldwin, J.A., Rolf, J.E., Johnson, J., Bowers, J., Benally, C., & Trotter, R.T. (1996). Developing culturally sensitive HIV/AIDS and substance abuse prevention curricula for Native American youth. *Journal of School Health, 66*, 322-327.

Benedict, S., Williams, R.D., & Hoomani, J. (1996). Method of discovery of breast cancer. *Cancer Practice, 4*, 147-155.

Brody, L.C., & Biesecker, B.B. (1998). Breast cancer susceptibility genes. BRCA1 and BRCA2. *Medicine, 77*, 208-226.

Bryan, A.D., Aiken, L.S., & West, S.G. (1997). Young women's condom use: The influence of responsibility for sexuality, control over the sexual encounter, and perceived susceptibility to common STDs. *Health Psychology, 16*, 468-479.

Busemeyer, J.R., & Jones, L. (1983). Analysis of multiplicative combination rules when the causal variables are measured with error. *Psychological Bulletin, 93*, 549-562.

Champion, V.L. (1990). Breast self examination in women 35 and older: A prospective study. *Journal of Behavioral Medicine, 13*(6), 523-538.

Champion, V.L., & Menon, U. (1997). Predicting mammography and breast self-examination in African American women. *Cancer Nursing, 20*(5), 315-322.

Champion, V.L., & Miller, T.K. (1992). Variables related to breast self-examination: Model generation. *Psychology of Women Quarterly, 16*, 81-96.

Champoux, J.E., & Peters, W.S. (1987). Form, effect size and power in moderated regression analysis. *Journal of Occupational Psychology, 60*, 243-255.

Clarke, V., Hill, D., Rassaby, J., White, V., & Hirst, S. (1991). Determinants of continued breast self examination practice in women 40 years and over after personalized instruction. *Health Education Research, 6*(3), 297-306.

Cohen, J. (1988). *Statistical power analysis for the behavioral sciences* (2nd ed.). Hillsdale, NJ: Lawrence Erlbaum.

Cope, D.G. (1992). Self-esteem and the practice of breast self-examination. *Western Journal of Nursing Research, 14*(5), 618-631.

Costanza, M.E. (1994). The extent of breast cancer screening in older women. *Cancer Supplement, 74*(7), 2046-2050.

Dijkstra, A., DeVries, H., Roijackers, J., & vanBreukelen, G. (1998). Tailored interventions to communicate stage-matched information to smokers in different motivational stages. *Journal of Consulting and Clinical Psychology, 66*, 549-557.

Duke, S.S., Gordon-Sosby, K., Reynolds, K.D., & Gram, I.T. (1994). A study of breast cancer detection practices and beliefs in Black women attending public health clinics. *Health Education Research, 9*, 331-342.

Fisher, J.D., & Fisher, W.A. (1992). Changing AIDS risk behavior. *Psychological Bulletin, 111*, 455-474.

Fisher, J.D., & Fisher, W.A. (2000). Theoretical approaches to individual-level change in HIV-risk behavior. In J. Peterson & R. DiClemente (Eds.), *HIV prevention handbook* (pp. 3-55). New York: Kluver Academic/Plenum.

Fletcher, S.W., Morgan, T.M., O'Malley, M.S., Earp, J.A., & Degnan, D. (1989). Is breast self-examination predicted by knowledge, attitudes, beliefs, or sociodemographic characteristics? *American Journal of Preventive Medicine, 5*, 207-215.

Fouad, M.N., Kiefe, C.I., Bartolucci, A.A., Burst, N.M., Ulene, V., & Harvey, M.R. (1997). A hypertension control program tailored to unskilled and minority workers. *Ethnicity and Disease, 7*, 191-199.

Friedman, L.C., Nelson, D.V., Webb, J.A., Hoffman, L.P., & Baer, P.E. (1994). Dispositional optimism, self-efficacy, and health beliefs as predictors of breast self-examination. *American Journal of Preventive Medicine, 10*, 130-135.

Gerrard, M., Gibbons, F.X., & Bushman, B.J. (1996). Relation between perceived vulnerability to HIV and precautionary sexual behavior. *Psychological Bulletin, 119*, 390-409.

Hailey, B.J., & Bradford, A.C. (1991). Breast self-examination and mammography among university staff and faculty. *Women and Health, 17*, 59-77.

Jaccard, J., Turrisi, R., & Wan, C.K. (1990). *Interaction effects in multiple regression*. Newbury Park: Sage.

Janz, N.K., & Becker, M.H. (1984). The Health Belief Model: A decade later. *Health Education Quarterly, 11*, 1-47.

King, E., Rimer, B.K., Benincasa, T., Harron, C., Amfoh, K., Bonney, G., Kornguth, P., Demark-Wahnefried, W., Strigo, T., & Engstrom, P. (1998). Strategies to encourage mammography use among women in senior citizens' housing facilities. *Journal of Cancer Education, 13*, 108-115.

King, T., Borrelli, B., Black, C., Pinto, B.M., & Marcus, B.H. (1997). Minority women and tobacco: Implications for smoking cessation interventions. *Annals of Behavioral Medicine, 19*, 310-313.

Lichtenstein, E. (1997). Behavioral research contributions and needs in cancer prevention and control: Tobacco use prevention and cessation. *Preventive Medicine, 26*, S57-63.

Lierman, L.M., Young, H.M., Kasprzyk, D., & Benoliel, J.Q. (1990). Predicting breast self-examination using the theory of reasoned action. *Nursing Research, 39*(2), 97-101.

Lu, Z. (1995). Variables associated with breast self-examination among Chinese women. *Cancer Nursing, 18*(1), 29-34.

Mamon, J., & Zapka, J.G. (1986). Breast self-examination by young women: I. Characteristics associated with frequency. *American Journal of Preventive Medicine, 2*, 61-69.

Maskarinec, G., Singh, S., Meng, L., & Franke, A.A. (1998). Dietary soy intake and urinary isoflavone excretion among women from a multiethnic population. *Cancer Epidemiology, Biomarkers, and Prevention, 7*, 613-619.

Massey, V. (1986). Perceived susceptibility to breast cancer and practice of breast self-examination. *Nursing Research, 35*, 183-185.

McClelland, G.H., & Judd, C.M. (1993). Statistical difficulties of detecting interactions and moderator effects. *Psychological Bulletin, 114*, 376-390.

McCoy, H.V., McCoy, C.B., & Lai, S. (1998). Effectiveness of HIV interventions among women drug users. *Women and Health, 27*, 49-66.

Mezzetti, M., La Vecchia, C., Decarli, A., Boyle, P., Talamini, R., & Franceschi, S. (1998). Population attributable risk for breast cancer: Diet, nutrition, and physical exercise. *Journal of the National Cancer Institute, 90*, 389-394.

Misovich, S.J., Fisher, J.D., Martinez, T., Bryan, A.D., & Catapano, N. (in review). Predicting breast self-examination: A test of the information, motivation, behavioral skills model of behavior change.

Perdue, P.W., Galbo, C., & Ghosh, B.C. (1995). Stratification of palpable and non-palpable breast cancer by method of detection and age. *Annals of Surgical Oncology, 2*, 512-515.

Pinto, B., & Fuqua, R.W. (1991). Training breast self-examination: A research review and critique. *Health Education Quarterly, 18*(4), 495-516.

Rassaby, J., Hirst, S., Hill, D.J., Bennett, R., & Clarke, V. (1991). Introduction of a breast self-examination teaching program in Victoria, Australia. *Health Education Research, 6*(3), 291-296.

Reeves, M.J., Newcomb, P.A., Remington, P.L., & Marcus, P.M. (1995). Determinants of breast cancer detection among Wisconsin (United States) women, 1988-90. *Cancer Causes and Control, 7*, 626-627.

Roche, M., & Gosnell, D. (1989). Evaluation of a hospital teaching program for breast self-examination. *Patient Education and Counseling, 13*, 31-41.

Ronis, D.L., & Kaiser, M.K. (1989). Correlates of breast self-examination in a sample of college women: Analyses of linear structural relations. *Journal of Applied Social Psychology, 19*(13), 1068-1084.

Ruda, P.A., Bourcier, F.M., & Skiff, D. (1992). Health beliefs of senior college students regarding breast cancer and breast self-examination. *Health Care for Women International, 13*, 33-41.

Salazar, M.K., Wilkinson, J.D., DeRoos, R.L., Lee, C.Y., Lyons, R., Rubadue, C., & Fetrick, A. (1994). Breast cancer behaviors following participation in a cancer risk appraisal. *Health Values, 18*(3), 41-49.

Senie, R.T., Lesser, R., Kinne, D.W., & Rosen, P.P. (1994). Method of tumor detection influences disease-free survival of women with breast carcinoma. *Cancer, 73*, 1666-1672.

Shepperd, S.L., Solomon, L.J., Atkins, E., Foster, R.S., Jr., & Frankowski, B. (1990). Determinants of breast self-examination among women of lower income and lower education. *Journal of Behavioral Medicine, 13*(4), 359-371.

Siero, S., Kok, G., & Pruyn, J. (1984). Effects of public education about breast cancer and breast self-examination. *Social Science and Medicine, 18*, 881-888.

Stillman, M.J. (1977). Women's health beliefs about breast cancer and breast self-examination. *Nursing Research, 26*(2), 121-127.

Strauss, L.M., Solomon, L.J., Costanza, M.C., Worden, J.K., & Foster, R.S., Jr. (1987). Breast self-examination practices and attitudes of women with and without a history of breast cancer. *Journal of Behavioral Medicine, 10*(4), 337-350.

Weinstein, N.D., & Nicolich, M. (1993). Correct and incorrect interpretations of correlations between risk perceptions and risk behaviors. *Health Psychology, 12,* 235-245.

Zedeck, S. (1971). Problems with the use of "moderator" variables. *Psychological Bulletin, 76,* 295-310.

Effectiveness
of a Cancer Education Program for Women Attending Rural Public Health Departments in North Carolina

Robert Michielutte
Louise E. Cunningham
Penny C. Sharp

Wake Forest University

Mark B. Dignan

University of Alabama at Birmingham

Virginia D. Burnette

Wake Forest University

Robert Michielutte, PhD, Louise E. Cunningham, MPH, Penny C. Sharp, EdD, and Virginia D. Burnette, BS, are affiliated with the Department of Family and Community Medicine, Wake Forest University School of Medicine, Winston-Salem, NC 27157.

Mark B. Dignan, PhD, is affiliated with the Department of Health and Behavior, University of Alabama at Birmingham, 1665 University Blvd., Suite 227, Birmingham, AL 35294.

Address correspondence to: Robert Michielutte, Wake Forest University School of Medicine, Department of Family and Community Medicine, Winston-Salem, NC 27157 (E-mail: *bmichiel@wfubmc.edu*).

This research was supported by grant R01-CA-60504 from the National Cancer Institute.

[Haworth co-indexing entry note]: "Effectiveness of a Cancer Education Program for Women Attending Rural Public Health Departments in North Carolina." Michielutte, Robert et al. Co-published simultaneously in *Journal of Prevention & Intervention in the Community* (The Haworth Press, Inc.) Vol. 22, No. 2, 2001, pp. 23-42; and: *Prevention Issues for Women's Health in the New Millennium* (ed: Wendee M. Wechsberg) The Haworth Press, Inc., 2001, pp. 23-42. Single or multiple copies of this article are available for a fee from The Haworth Document Delivery Service [1-800-342-9678, 9:00 a.m. - 5:00 p.m. (EST). E-mail address: getinfo@haworthpressinc.com].

© 2001 by The Haworth Press, Inc. All rights reserved.

SUMMARY. The Western North Carolina Cancer Awareness Program (CAP) was a four-year program, funded by the National Cancer Institute, to increase education and support services for the prevention and early detection of breast, cervical, and skin cancer among women receiving care in six rural county public health departments. Three health departments were selected as intervention units, and the remaining three health departments served as comparison units. Women age 20 and older were randomly selected in each health department. Women in the intervention group received a comprehensive health education program that included easy-to-read printed materials and telephone counseling dealing with breast, cervical, and skin cancer. Theoretical guidelines for development of the intervention program included the PRECEDE Model and the Health Belief Model. Overall, the results indicated that personalized education, which includes the combination of readable printed materials and telephone contact, can be effective in increasing some early detection behaviors for breast and skin cancer among women who attend public health departments. The value of telephone counseling as a comparatively inexpensive approach to individualizing health education has significant implications for the development of similar cancer education programs for underserved populations. *[Article copies available for a fee from The Haworth Document Delivery Service: 1-800-342-9678. E-mail address: <getinfo@haworthpressinc. com> Website: <http://www.HaworthPress. com> © 2001 by The Haworth Press, Inc. All rights reserved.]*

KEYWORDS. Breast cancer, cervical cancer, skin cancer, cancer education, public health, rural

One of the most consistent findings in the literature on health and illness is the negative association between social class and illness. Regardless of the way in which social class is defined, several decades of research have found that lower social class is associated with a greater risk of disease incidence, mortality, and morbidity (Syme & Berkman, 1989; Feinstein, 1993; Marmot & Feeney, 1997). With some exceptions, lower social class also is associated with higher incidence, morbidity, and mortality from cancer (Linden, 1969; Lipworth, Abelin, & Connelly, 1970; Berg, Ross, & LaTourette, 1977; Freeman, 1989; Kogevinas & Porta, 1997; Faggiano, Partanen, Kogevinas, & Boffetta, 1997) and with lower participation in cancer prevention and early detection programs (Katz & Hofer, 1994; Anderson & May, 1995; Ruchlin, 1997; Hiatt & Pasick, 1996; Segnan, 1997; Hoffman-Goetz, Breen, & Meissner, 1998; Hall, May, Lew, Koh, & Nadel, 1997).

Inner-city residents, minorities, the elderly, and rural residents constitute a large proportion of the nation's poor. In addition, while urban populations have documented higher incidence and mortality rates from cancer (Liff, Chow, & Greenberg, 1991), rural populations have generally less favorable health status (Braden & Beauregard, 1994). Cancer patients in rural areas are diagnosed at later stages of the disease and have a larger proportion of unstaged cancers at the time of diagnosis (Liff, Chow, & Greenberg, 1991; Monroe, Ricketts, & Savitz, 1992). Rural populations are more likely to a have a larger percentage of individuals with lower income and education, and they usually have a larger elderly population (Liff, Chow, & Greenberg, 1991; Summer, 1991; Miller, Stokes, & Clifford, 1987). Rural populations also have poorer access to health care services, fewer cancer prevention activities, and less receptivity to health resources (Liff, Chow, & Greenberg, 1991; Braden & Beauregard, 1994).

In general, the available information suggests that increased attention should be directed to the development of cancer control programs in rural areas, particularly targeted to the lower socioeconomic subgroups in the population. Development of successful interventions to increase accessibility to information on cancer prevention, early detection, and treatment for low-income, low-education individuals at higher risk of cancer should be given high priority.

THE PRESENT STUDY

To address this void, the National Cancer Institute (NCI) funded the Western North Carolina Cancer Awareness Program (CAP), a community-based cancer control program. The general objective of the program was to develop, implement, and evaluate a cancer prevention and early detection program based in rural public health departments. The program's goals were to: (a) increase women's knowledge of skin, breast, and cervical cancer; (b) encourage positive attitudes toward cancer prevention and early detection; (c) increase the number of women who obtain clinical skin exams, Pap smears, clinical breast exams, and mammograms; and (d) increase the number of women who practice skin cancer prevention, skin self-exam, and breast self-exam.

The intervention program was designed to effect changes within the health departments with regard to cancer control activities, as well as to test a specific educational approach for individual women. A comprehensive description of the program, including the results dealing with the health department as the unit of the analysis, has been published elsewhere (Cunningham, Michielutte, Dignan, Sharp, & Boxley, 2000). This article presents the results of the intervention targeted to individual women.

METHODS

Background

PRECEDE-PROCEED Model. Identification of the barriers to early detection and prevention of cancer followed the framework set forth in the PRECEDE-PROCEED Model (Green, Krueter, & Deeds, 1980; Green & Krueter, 1991). PRECEDE is an approach to health education planning that incorporates elements of the health belief model, social learning theory, and a number of general models of health behavior. PRECEDE is an acronym that stands for "predisposing, reinforcing, and enabling causes in educational diagnosis and evaluation" (Green, Krueter, & Deeds, 1980). Rather than beginning with the design of a health education program, the PRECEDE model begins with a consideration of social problems associated with quality of life and works backward to identification of specific health problems that contribute to these social problems. The next phase consists of identifying health-related behaviors that seem to be associated with the health problem to be addressed, which in turn leads to a consideration of factors that might affect these health behaviors.

The three types of issues considered in the model are predisposing, enabling, and reinforcing factors. Predisposing factors consist of attitudes, values, beliefs, and perceptions that facilitate or hinder personal motivation for change. Absence of enabling factors represents potential barriers created by societal forces or systems: for example, limited medical facilities, inadequate personal resources, restrictive laws, lack of health insurance, or lack of knowledge required for the desired behavioral change. Reinforcing factors consist of feedback, both negative and positive, from others that contribute to specific behaviors.

Once information on all elements of the model is specified and the necessary diagnostic information is obtained with respect to the impact of the three classes of factors, it is possible to develop, implement, and evaluate health education programs based on the relative importance of different factors and the different resources available to influence them (the PROCEED process).

One of the first steps in developing the CAP program dealt with identification and elaboration of these factors among women in the target population through information obtained in the baseline interviews. An understanding of predisposing, enabling, and reinforcing factors affecting cancer prevention and early detection activities in the target communities helped guide development of the educational messages for women.

Health Belief Model. The Health Belief Model was also used in the intervention design as a guide to development of the specific content of the messages. This model assumes that individuals fear illness and that the likelihood of taking health actions in response to illness is associated with the degree of fear and the expected fear-reduction potential of actions, as long as the perceived benefits outweigh the practical and psychological obstacles to taking these actions (Glanz & Rimer, 1995). The constructs of the Health Belief Model in its present form include perceived susceptibility, perceived severity, perceived benefits, perceived barriers, cues to action, and self-efficacy. As Glanz and Rimer noted, the Health Belief Model can be an effective mechanism for guiding the development of persuasive messages for health actions such as screening mammography. Information obtained in the context of PRECEDE-PROCEED provided guidelines for dealing with both barriers and facilitators to cancer screening that were directly applicable to the elements of the Health Belief Model. This information was used to develop messages that were designed to be both informative and persuasive with regard to participation in breast, cervical, and skin cancer screening and prevention activities.

Intervention Approaches. Several health education approaches designed for cancer control have met with varying degrees of success. To determine the most effective intervention approach, we reviewed over 50 recent publications reporting the results of programs to increase cancer control activities and found that the most common approaches included mass media messages, printed educational materials, direct education using professional or lay health educators, and telephone counseling. Many programs, especially community-based projects, used various combinations of these approaches. Personal contact with program participants through direct education generally was the most effective approach, but also was the most expensive and time-consuming. Printed educational materials can be effective, but generally are most valuable when used in combination with other educational approaches. One problem with printed materials is that, when program participants are members of underserved populations (low-income, low-education, minority, elderly), a fairly large proportion of the population is likely to be functionally illiterate or have low literacy skills.

Telephone counseling has been found to be an effective educational approach that involves personal contact, while being much less expensive than direct, face-to-face education. Soet and Basch (1997) note several advantages of the telephone as a means of communication for health education. Telephone contact is interactive and allows direct participation of the individual in the program. It is less stressful in that visual privacy can reduce stress and make the communication more productive. It is less costly and less time consuming than face-to-face contact and, because of the lower cost, educators can make more frequent contacts. Finally, it can broaden the scope of the audience a program can reach. Educators can bring the program to dispersed populations such as those in rural areas, homebound populations, and low-literacy populations that may not be able to get the needed information from written materials.

Soet and Basch (1997) also point out a number of disadvantages of the telephone in health education. In telephone contact, nonverbal cues are lost, the communication may seem impersonal or anonymous, participants may prefer visual learning over auditory learning, and a program based only on telephone contact will exclude those without telephones or who have handicaps such as hearing disabilities. Despite these limitations, Soet and Basch (1997) conclude that research to date suggests that using the telephone as a means of educational intervention is a promising approach to health education for behavior change.

The Intervention Program

Based on the results of previous studies, the intervention program selected for individual women in the present scenario was a combination of printed educational materials and telephone counseling. All educational materials and the telephone counseling script were pilot tested with small samples of women from the intervention health departments. Intervention activities were coordinated by project health educators based in each health department. Two health educators delivered the intervention during the initial evaluation period. One was based in Clay County, and one split her time between Henderson and Transylvania Counties.

Women participating in the program were sent mailings of educational literature on breast, cervical, and skin cancer at two-month intervals. The printed educational literature included what we found to be the most readable of existing materials on breast, cervical, and skin cancer, as well as fact sheets developed by project staff. The printed materials had readability levels that ranged between 5th and 8th grade, as measured by the Flesch-Kincaid formula (Ley & Florio, 1996).

A follow-up telephone counseling call was made to all women who could be reached by the health educator to answer questions and address any barriers to the recommended prevention and screening activities. After the telephone calls took place, a final mailing was sent that included a fact sheet reinforcing key points regarding breast, cervical, and skin cancer. In this mailing, the women were given the opportunity to participate in a contest for gift certificates for groceries by answering three prevention and early detection questions on a postcard and returning the card to enter the contest. To maintain contact with women from health departments in the comparison counties, as well as to provide them with some educational information, they were sent one mailing of print materials dealing with nutrition and cancer. They did not receive telephone counseling calls.

Process Evaluation

A detailed process evaluation was conducted during the course of the CAP project to monitor implementation, identify problems, and develop specific solutions. Prior to beginning the educational program, the two project health educators completed a workshop dealing with all components of the intervention, including the educational materials to be used and the telephone counseling script. Their activities were monitored on a weekly basis for the duration of the project.

Components of the process evaluation included documentation of project activities, feedback from health department staff, and feedback from women who participated in the program. Program documentation and review were conducted for materials development, distribution of printed materials, the telephone follow-up, weekly health educator activities, correspondence, and data collection activities. A 10% quality-control check of interviews with participants was conducted for both pretest and posttest surveys. A detailed description of the process evaluation procedures used in the CAP project, the results, and the subsequent program modifications (or simply recognition of the problems when no modifications were possible) are described in Cunningham et al. (2000).

Outcome Evaluation

The research design for the evaluation was a quasi-experimental design in which the six participating health departments were assigned to intervention and comparison groups. As previously noted, the program was directed to both the health departments and to individual women. Thus, some components of the educational program were available to all women served by the health departments, and randomization of women within each health department to intervention and comparison groups was not an option.

Prior to selection of the participating health departments, counties in western North Carolina were classified and matched according to size, percent urban, per capita income, percent minority population, geographical proximity, and characteristics of the health departments. The six counties selected for the study formed three roughly matched pairs, consisting of two very small, all rural counties (Clay and Alleghany, populations < 10,000), two somewhat larger counties (Transylvania and Alexander, populations 25,000 to 30,000), and two moderately large counties (Henderson and Burke, populations 69,000 to 76,000). All of the counties have over a 93% Caucasian resident population. Within each pair, the health departments provided similar services to their clients.

Interaction between the staff of the six participating health departments was a possible contaminating factor in evaluating the program. To minimize this interaction, the counties were selected to allow two similar groupings in different geographical locations. While the assignment to geographical groupings was nonrandom, selection of the group of counties to receive the intervention was done randomly. Clay, Transylvania, and Henderson Counties formed a natural geographic cluster in the far western corner of North Carolina, and their health departments were selected to receive the program. Alleghany, Alexander, and Burke Counties are located in west-central North Carolina, and their health departments were selected for the comparison group. Following the initial evaluation period (1994-1996) to be described in this article, all health departments participated in program activities (1996-1997).

Evaluation of the intervention was conducted by comparing pretest and posttest self-reports of breast, cervical, and skin cancer prevention and early detection behaviors. Female clients of the health departments age 20 and older, who were residents of the county and who indicated they did not plan to move from the county in the next year, were eligible for the study. All women recruited for the study either had a telephone at the time of the initial interview or had access to one through a neighbor. Age 20 was selected as the lower age limit for participation to include women eligible for all screening tests, with the exception of mammography, based on current American Cancer Society guidelines. Evaluation of mammography screening was limited to women age 40 and older.

Women attending the health department were recruited by randomly sampling waiting room locations (based on a map of chairs in each waiting room) during scheduled clinics. Baseline face-to-face interviews were completed with 1180 eligible women in the six health departments, representing approximately 70% of the women approached. Information obtained in the interviews included social and demographic information, health status, knowledge of risk factors for the cancers of interest, perceived barriers to screening, and current screening behavior for breast, cervical, and skin cancer. The women also provided information on skin cancer prevention.

Preliminary analyses of the baseline data revealed no significant differences between women in the program and comparison groups except for age. The age distributions showed a larger proportion of women age 50 and older in the intervention group and a larger proportion of women age 20-29 in the comparison group.

Approximately 14 months later, posttest interviews were completed by telephone with 749 women, representing 63.5% of the eligible women surveyed at baseline. A comparison of responders and nonresponders to the posttest survey revealed that they differed significantly only by age. Younger women were more likely to be lost to follow-up. More importantly, the characteristics of women lost to follow-up were similar for both the intervention and comparison groups. Background characteristics of women in the intervention and comparison groups who completed both the pretest and posttest surveys are shown in Table 1. The significant age differential observed in the total pretest sample is maintained, but the two groups are similar in all other background characteristics.

The outcome behaviors were having had: (a) a cervical smear, (b) a clinical breast exam, or (c) a mammogram in the past year (women over 40 years old); (d) a clinical skin exam (ever); (e) at least one skin self-exam in the past year; (f) a monthly breast self-exam; and (g) the use of sunscreen when outdoors for an extended period of time in the spring and summer. All outcomes were examined as dichotomies (0-NO, 1-YES).

Statistical Analysis

Cluster sampling was used to select the study sample. A nonrandom assignment to intervention and comparison groups was made at the health department level. Sample selection was done randomly within each health department, and the analysis was conducted using the individual woman as the unit of analysis. Murray and Wolfinger (1994) have noted that the observations for individuals within the larger assignment units will be correlated due to common experiences and/or other selection factors. Under these circumstances, analysis of the outcomes using individuals as the unit of analysis can result in a badly inflated Type I error, resulting in a greater chance of erroneously concluding that the intervention program is successful. They emphasize that, when conducting the analysis at the individual level, one must be able to include the assignment units as nested random effects in the analysis in order to achieve the desired Type I error rate.

Tests for the two-way tabulations comparing the intervention and comparison groups that take into account the cluster sampling design were conducted using an adjustment to the usual Pearson chi-square statistic. This adjustment is based on a second order Rao and Scott correction that results in an "F" statistic. This statistic has a probability distribution that can be interpreted in the same way as the distribution for chi-square based on simple random sampling (StataCorp, 1999).

Multiple logistic regression analysis for binary dependent variables was used to test for the significance of intervention and comparison posttest group differences, adjusting for the pretest scores and background characteristics of the women. The adjustment for cluster sampling in the regression analyses was made using robust variance estimators for clustered data provided in the STATA statistical software package (StataCorp, 1999). In addition to controlling for age, tests for potential confounding variables included controlling for each of the characteristics of the women shown in Table 1. Education, health insurance, and race were found to affect the association between group (intervention vs. comparison) and the outcome variables, and they were included in the final analyses.

RESULTS

Pretest and posttest outcome scores for the intervention and comparison groups are shown in Table 2. Women in the intervention group reported larger percentages engaging in each cancer control activity after they completed the intervention program. The largest changes were for clinical skin exam (+17 percentage points) and breast self-exam (+11 percentage points). With the exception of clinical breast exam (− 2 percentage points), changes in cancer control behaviors reported by women in the comparison group also were positive, with the largest change being for clinical skin exam (+14 percentage points). As would be expected if the intervention were successful, the increases in all cancer screening and prevention behaviors from pretest to posttest are greater for women in the intervention group. However, as shown in the last column of Table 2, the net advantage for the intervention group is 3 percentage points or less for all behaviors except breast self-exam (+8 percentage points).

Table 3 shows the formal test for intervention effects controlling for age (and other characteristics of the women) and adjusting for pretest scores. These data indicate significantly greater odds of women in the intervention group practicing breast self-exam (p = 0.003) and getting a clinical skin exam (p = 0.024) and marginal significance for getting a clinical breast exam (p = 0.073). The results are not significant for the other cancer-control behaviors.

An additional factor to be considered in evaluating the intervention is that a fairly large number of women in the intervention group did not receive the telephone counseling component of the program. Many women in the participating health departments tend to have their telephones disconnected and reconnected at different times. Of the 384 women in the intervention group, 116 (30%) could not be reached during the telephone counseling period; but they could be reached later at the time of the posttest interview. Similarly, about 20% of the

TABLE 1. Characteristics of Women in the Intervention and Comparison Groups

	Intervention		Comparison		F^a	p-value
	N	%	N	%		
Number of Women	384[b]		365[b]			
Age					4.85	0.047
20–24	47	12.3	94	25.8		
25–29	55	14.3	76	20.8		
30–49	140	36.4	148	40.5		
50–64	68	17.7	30	8.2		
65 or older	74	19.3	17	4.7		
Head of Household					<0.01	0.989
No	273	72.2	261	72.3		
Yes	105	27.8	100	27.7		
Marital Status					0.01	0.917
Married/Living Together	278	73.2	261	72.7		
Other	102	26.8	99	27.3		
Health Insurance					0.17	0.701
Private/Medicare	212	55.9	217	59.9		
None/Medicaid	167	44.1	145	40.1		
Education					0.88	0.443
11th Grade or Less	86	22.6	83	22.9		
High School/GED/ Technical	182	47.9	147	40.6		
Some College/ Jr College	73	19.2	85	23.5		
4-Year College Degree	39	10.3	47	13.0		
Race					3.72	0.112
White	370	96.4	331	90.9		
Black/Asian	14	3.6	33	9.1		

[a]Pearson chi-square statistic adjusted for cluster sampling using the second-order.
Rao and Scott Correction (StataCorp, 1999).
[b]Sample sizes differ slightly for each variable due to missing information.

women who received the telephone counseling could not be contacted for the posttest interview. Tests for potential bias based on the pretest data did not reveal any significant background differences between women in the intervention group who did and did not receive telephone counseling (Table 4). Therefore, after conducting the basic tests

TABLE 2. Changes in Cancer Control Outcomes After Completion of the Intervention Program

	Percent Who Responded Yes						
	Intervention Group (N = 384)[a]			Comparison Group (N = 365)[a]			Difference
Cancer Screening/ Prevention Activity	Pretest	Post-test	Change, I_c	Pretest	Post-test	Change, C_c	$I_c - C_c$
Pap Smear in Past Year	66	68	+2	71	72	+1	+1
Mammogram in Past Year (Women 40+)[b]	51	55	+4	43	44	+1	+3
Clinical Breast Exam in Past Year	69	70	+1	70	68	−2	+3
Monthly Breast Self Exam	56	67	+11	55	58	+3	+8
Ever Had Clinical Skin Exam	23	40	+17	15	29	+14	+3
At Least One Skin Self Exam in Past Year	30	44	+14	23	36	+13	+1
Always Use Sunscreen in Spring and Summer	29	34	+5	35	37	+2	+3

[a]Sample sizes differ slightly for each outcome due to missing information.
[b]Sample sizes for women 40 and older are N = 193 for the intervention group; N = 95 for the comparison group.

for program effects, the intervention group was split into "print only" and "print plus telephone counseling."

The multivariate analysis shown in Table 3 was repeated using the expanded definition of the intervention group. This analysis contrasted the print only and print plus telephone counseling groups with the comparison group (Table 5). The adjusted odds ratios (AOR) revealed that the differences in favor of the intervention group were stronger in the print plus telephone counseling group for breast self-exam (print only AOR = 1.32, p = 0.128; print plus telephone AOR = 1.67, p < .001) and for clinical skin exam (print only AOR = 0.66, p = 0.126; print plus telephone AOR = 1.65, p = 0.001). Although the adjusted odds ratios were not significant for either group, the same pattern of differences was found for mammography (print only AOR = 1.05, p = .783; print plus telephone AOR = 1.65, p = 0.069), and for skin self-

TABLE 3. Multivariate Logistic Regression Analysis of Posttest Cancer Control Outcomes, Comparison vs. Total Intervention Group

Cancer Control Screening or Prevention Activity	N[a]	AOR[b]	95% CI	p-value
Pap Smear in Past Year				
Intervention	376	1.03	0.79,1.34	0.836
Comparison	359	1.00		
Mammogram in Past Year (Women 40 and Older)				
Intervention	191	1.48	0.86, 2.54	0.155
Comparison	95	1.00		
Clinical Breast Exam in Past Year				
Intervention	374	1.31	0.98,1.77	0.073
Comparison	361	1.00		
Performed Monthly Breast Self-Exam				
Intervention	375	1.55	1.16, 2.08	0.003
Comparison	359	1.00		
Ever Had Clinical Skin Exam				
Intervention	376	1.32	1.04, 1.68	0.024
Comparison	360	1.00		
At Least One Skin Self-Exam				
Intervention	378	1.21	0.75, 1.94	0.434
Comparison	360	1.00		
Always Use Sunscreen in Spring and Summer				
Intervention	378	0.88	0.54, 1.42	0.596
Comparison	361	1.00		

[a]Number of women in the intervention and comparison groups.
[b]Comparison group is the reference group. Adjusted odds ratios (AOR) are adjusted for age, race, education, health insurance, and pretest scores. Variance estimates for the confidence intervals and p-levels adjusted for cluster sampling (StataCorp, 1999).

exam (print only AOR = 0.86, p = 0.674; print plus telephone AOR = 1.40, p = .148). Cervical screening, clinical breast exam, and sunscreen use showed only small and inconsistent differences by intervention group. Again the results are mixed, but they reinforce the importance of telephone contact.

CONCLUSION

This study tested the value of an educational program using low-literacy printed materials and follow-up telephone counseling to in-

TABLE 4. Characteristics of Women in the Print Only and Print Plus Telephone Counseling Intervention Groups

| | Intervention Group | | | | | |
| | Print Only | | Print + Telephone | | | |
	N	%	N	%	F^a	p-value
Number of Women	116[b]		268[b]			
Age					0.31	0.655
20-24	20	17.2	27	10.1		
25-29	18	15.5	37	13.8		
30-49	34	29.3	106	39.6		
50-64	28	24.1	40	14.9		
65 or older	16	13.8	58	21.6		
Head of Household					0.09	0.797
No	80	70.8	193	72.8		
Yes	33	29.2	72	27.2		
Marital Status					2.21	0.275
Married/Living Together	75	65.2	203	76.6		
Other	40	34.7	62	23.4		
Health Insurance					0.19	0.708
Private/Medicare	61	53.5	151	56.9		
None/Medicaid	53	46.5	114	43.0		
Education					1.01	0.431
11th Grade or Less	28	24.3	58	21.9		
High School/GED/ Technical	61	53.0	121	45.7		
Some College/ Jr College	16	13.9	57	21.5		
4-Year College Degree	10	8.7	29	10.9		
Race					3.22	0.215
White	111	95.6	259	96.6		
Black/Asian	5	4.3	9	3.3		

[a]Pearson chi-square statistic adjusted for cluster sampling using the second-order
Rao and Scott Correction (StataCorp, 1999).

crease prevention and screening for breast, cervical, and skin cancer in a population of women served by rural health departments. The evaluation had some methodological deficiencies that limit generalization of the results. The study design assigned intervention and control units at the health department level but sampled and conducted the evaluation using the individual woman as the unit of analysis. The interven-

TABLE 5. Multivariate Logistic Regression Analysis of Posttest Cancer Control Outcomes, Comparison vs. Print Materials Only and Print Materials Plus Telephone Counseling Intervention Groups

Cancer Control Screening or Prevention Activity	N[a]	AOR[b]	95% CI	p-value
Pap Smear in Past Year				
Print Only	112	0.93	0.67, 1.30	0.686
Print + Telephone	264	1.07	0.83, 1.38	0.578
Comparison	359	1.00		
Mammogram in Past Year (Women 40 and Older)				
Print Only	50	1.06	0.72, 1.56	0.783
Print + Telephone	141	1.65	0.96, 2.84	0.069
Comparison	95	1.00		
Clinical Breast Exam in Past Year				
Print Only	110	1.38	1.04, 1.83	0.026
Print + Telephone	264	1.28	0.95, 1.74	0.103
Comparison	361	1.00		
Performed Monthly Breast Self-Exam				
Print Only	111	1.32	0.92, 1.89	0.134
Print + Telephone	264	1.67	1.27, 2.21	<0.001
Comparison	359	1.00		
Ever Had Clinical Skin Exam				
Print Only	112	1.04	0.75, 1.46	0.798
Print + Telephone	264	1.45	1.16, 1.82	0.001
Comparison	360	1.00		
At Least One Skin Self-Exam				
Print Only	113	0.86	0.42, 1.75	0.674
Print + Telephone	265	1.40	0.89, 2.20	0.148
Comparison	360	1.00		
Always Use Sunscreen in Spring and Summer				
Print Only	114	1.00	0.45, 2.24	0.996
Print + Telephone	264	0.82	0.56, 1.22	0.333
Comparison	361	1.00		

[a]Number of women in the intervention and comparison groups.
[b]Comparison group is the reference group. Adjusted odds ratios (AOR) are adjusted for age, race, education, health insurance, and pretest scores. Variance estimates for the confidence intervals and p-levels adjusted for cluster sampling (StataCorp, 1997).

tion and control groups were nonequivalent with regard to age, and several other potentially confounding factors also had to be controlled in the analysis. Follow-up of women was difficult, and only about two-thirds of the women who initially enrolled in the study could be reached for the posttest interview. However, examination of the pretest data indicated that, except for age, women lost to follow-up were similar to the women contacted during the posttest period. In addition, our experience with telephone disconnects and reconnects and the general mobility of younger health department clients suggested that no serious biases were introduced by the low follow-up rate.

Despite these limitations, the results support the conclusion that personalized education, which includes the combination of readable printed materials and telephone contact, can be effective in increasing some early detection behaviors for breast and skin cancer among women who attend public health departments. Further analysis of the data splitting the intervention group into print only and print plus telephone counseling also suggests the hypothesis that readable printed materials alone may not be sufficient to increase cancer prevention and early detection.

The present study supports earlier research that reported successful use of telephone contact for health education. In the area of cancer control, telephone counseling has been used together with printed materials in smoking cessation programs (Curry, McBride, Grothaus, Louie, & Wagner, 1995; Orleans et al., 1991), skin cancer screening (Mullan, Gardiner, Rosenman, Zhu, & Swanson, 1996), and mammography screening (King, Ross, Seay, Balsheim, & Rimer, 1995; Rimer, Ross, Balsheim, & Engstrom, 1993; Davis et al., 1997). Davis et al. (1997) also found that telephone contact plus a birthday card reminder was more effective than the birthday card reminder alone, or a combination of the card, a physician letter, and educational materials. Focusing more specifically on low-income populations, telephone counseling interventions have been successful in improving cervical and mammography screening (Lantz et al., 1995) and in increasing follow-up for abnormal cervical smears (Miller et al., 1997).

Telephone counseling is a promising health education approach that merits further attention as a means of improving cancer prevention and early detection in high-risk populations. A growing body of research, including the present study, supports its potential effectiveness. However, as demonstrated in the present study, an important limitation of this approach is the likelihood that a comparatively large proportion of individuals will be difficult to reach by telephone when dealing with low-income, underserved populations. Our experience suggests that the most effective use of telephone counseling as a health education strategy for underserved populations will be to incorporate it as only one component of a comprehensive individualized approach that also includes face-to-face contact in a clinic/practice setting and, when necessary, in the individual's home.

REFERENCES

Anderson, L.M., & May, D.S. (1995). Has the use of cervical, breast, and colorectal screening increased in the United States? *American Journal of Public Health, 85,* 840-842.

Berg, J.W., Ross, R., & LaTourette, H.B. (1977). Economic status and survival of cancer patients. *Cancer, 39,* 467-477.

Braden, J., & Beauregard, K. (1994). Health status and access to care of rural and urban populations. ACHPR Publication No. 94-0031. National Medical Expenditure Findings 18. Agency for Health Care Policy and Research. Rockville, MD: Public Health Service.

Cunningham, L.E., Michielutte, R., Dignan, M., Sharp, P., & Boxley, J. (2000). The value of process evaluation in a community-based cancer control program. *Evaluation and Program Planning, 23,* 13-25.

Curry, S.J., McBride, C., Grothaus, L.C., Louie, D., & Wagner, E.H. (1995). A randomized trial of self-help materials, personalized feedback, and telephone counseling with non-volunteer smokers. *Journal of Consulting and Clinical Psychology, 63,* 1005-1014.

Davis, N.A., Nash, E., Bailey, C., Lewis, M.J., Rimer, B.K., & Koplan, J.P. (1997). Evaluation of three methods for improving mammography rates in a managed care plan. *American Journal of Preventive Medicine, 13,* 298-302.

Faggiano, F., Partanen, T., Kogevinas, M., & Boffetta, P. (1997). Socioeconomic differences in cancer incidence and mortality. In M. Kogevinas, N. Pearce, M. Susser, & P. Boffetta (Eds.), *Social inequalities and cancer,* pp. 69-85. IARC Scientific Publications No. 138. Lyon: International Agency for Research on Cancer.

Feinstein, J.S. (1993). The relationship between socioeconomic status and health: A review of the literature. *Milbank Quarterly, 71,* 279-322.

Freeman, H.P. (1989). Cancer in the socioeconomically disadvantaged. *CA-A Cancer Journal for Clinicians, 38,* 266-288.

Glanz, K., & Rimer, B.K. (1995). *Theory at a glance: A guide for health promotion practice.* NIH Publication No. 95-3896. Washington, DC: U.S. Department of Health and Human Services, Public Health Service, National Institutes of Health, July.

Green, L.W., & Krueter, M.W. (1991). *Health promotion planning: An educational and environmental approach* (2nd ed.). Mountain View, CA: Mayfield Publishing Company.

Green, L.W., Krueter, M.W., & Deeds, S.G. (1980). *Health education planning: A diagnostic approach.* Palo Alto: Mayfield Publishing Company.

Hall, H.I., May, D.S., Lew, R.A., Koh, H.K., & Nadel, M. (1997). Sun protection behaviors of the U.S. white population. *Preventive Medicine, 26,* 401-407.

Hiatt, R.A., & Pasick, R.J. (1996). Unsolved problems in early breast cancer detection: Focus on the underserved. *Breast Cancer Research and Treatment, 40,* 37-51.

Hoffman-Goetz, L., Breen, N.L., & Meissner, H. (1998). The impact of social class on the use of cancer screening within three racial/ethnic groups in the United States. *Ethnicity and Disease, 8,* 3-51.

Katz, S.J., & Hofer, T.P. (1994). Socioeconomic disparities in preventive care persist despite universal coverage: Breast and cervical cancer screening in Ontario and the United States. *Journal of the American Medical Association, 272,* 530-534.

King, E.S., Ross, E., Seay, J., Balsheim, A., & Rimer, B. (1995). Mammography interventions for 65-74 year-old HMO women: Program effectiveness and predictors of use. *Journal of Aging and Health, 7,* 529-551.

Kogevinas, M., & Porta, M. (1997). Socioeconomic differences in cancer survival: A review of the evidence. In M. Kogevinas, N. Pearce, M. Susser, & P. Boffetta (Eds.), *Social inequalities and cancer,* pp. 177-206. IARC Scientific Publications No. 138. Lyon: International Agency for Research on Cancer.

Lantz, P.M., Stencil, D., Lippert, M.T., Beversdorf, S., Jaros, L., & Remington, P.L. (1995). Breast and cervical cancer screening in a low-income managed care sample: The efficacy of physician letters and phone calls. *American Journal of Public Health, 85,* 834-836.

Ley, P., & Florio, T. (1996). The use of readability formulas in health care. *Psychology, Health & Medicine, 1,* 7-28.

Liff, J.M., Chow, W.H., & Greenberg, W.S. (1991). Rural-urban differences in stage at diagnosis: Possible relationship to cancer screening. *Cancer, 67,* 1454-1459.

Linden, G. (1969). The influence of social class in the survival of cancer patients. *American Journal of Public Health, 59,* 267-274.

Lipworth, L., Abelin, T., & Connelly, R.R. (1970). Socio-economic factors in the prognosis of cancer patients. *Journal of Chronic Diseases, 23,* 105-115.

Marmot, M., & Feeney, A. (1997). General explanations for social inequalities in health. In M. Kogevinas, N. Pearce, M. Susser, & P. Boffetta (Eds.), *Social inequalities and cancer,* pp. 207-228. IARC Scientific Publications No. 138. Lyon: International Agency for Research on Cancer.

Miller, M.K., Stokes, C.S., & Clifford, W.B. (1987). A comparison of the rural-urban mortality differential for deaths from all causes, cardiovascular disease, and cancer. *Journal of Rural Health, 3,* 23-34.

Miller, S.M., Siejak, K.K., Schroeder, C.M., Lerman, C., Hernandez, E., & Helm, C.W. (1997). Enhancing adherence following abnormal Pap smears among low-income minority women: A preventive telephone counseling strategy. *Journal of the National Cancer Institute, 89,* 703-708.

Monroe, A.C., Ricketts, T.C., & Savitz, L.A. (1992). Cancer in rural versus urban populations: A review. *Journal of Rural Health, 8,* 212-220.

Mullan, P.B., Gardiner, J.C., Rosenman, K., Zhu, Z., & Swanson, G.M. (1996). Skin cancer prevention and detection practices in a Michigan farm population following an educational intervention. *Journal of Rural Health, 12,* 311-320.

Murray, D.M., & Wolfinger, R.D. (1994). Analysis issues in the evaluation of community trials: Progress toward solutions in SAS/STAT MIXED. *Journal of Community Psychology, CSAP, Special Issue*, 140-154.

Orleans, C.T., Schoenback, V.J., Wagner, E.H., Quade, D., Salmon, M.A., Pearson, D.C., Fiedler, J., Porter, C.O., & Kaplan, B.H. (1991). Effects of self-help materials, social support instructions, and telephone counseling. *Journal of Consulting and Clinical Psychology, 59*, 439-448.

Rimer, B.K., Ross, E., Balsheim, A., & Engstrom, P.F. (1993). The effect of a comprehensive breast cancer screening program on self-reported mammography use by primary care physicians and women in a health maintenance organization. *Journal of the American Board of Family Practice, 6*, 443-451.

Ruchlin, H.S. (1997). Prevalence and correlates of breast and cervical cancer screening among older women. *Obstetrics and Gynecology, 90*, 16-21.

Segnan, N. (1997). Socioeconomic status and cancer screening. In M. Kogevinas, N. Pearce, M. Susser, & P. Boffetta (Eds.), *Social inequalities and cancer*, pp. 369-376. IARC Scientific Publications No. 138. Lyon: International Agency for Research on Cancer.

Soet, J., & Basch, C.E. (1997). The telephone as a communication medium for health education. *Health Education & Behavior, 24*, 759-772.

StataCorp (1999). *Stata Statistical Software: Release 6.0*. College Station, TX: Stata Corporation.

Summer, L. (1991). Limited access, health care for the rural poor. *Center on Budget and Policy Priorities*, March.

Syme, S.L., & Berkman, L.F. (1989). Social class, susceptibility, and sickness. In H.D. Schwartz & C.S. Kart (Eds.), *Dominant issues in medical sociology*, pp. 398-405. Reading, MA: Addison-Wesley.

The Influence of Sexual Orientation on Health Behaviors in Women

Diane Powers
Fred Hutchinson Cancer Research Center

Deborah J. Bowen
University of Washington

Jocelyn White
Legacy Good Samaritan Medical Center

SUMMARY. Lesbians may be at risk for poorer health outcomes than heterosexual women because of differential health behaviors and risk factors for disease. Difficulty recruiting representative lesbian populations and a lack of simple, accurate measures of sexual orientation have hindered research about the differential health risks and outcomes faced by lesbian and heterosexual women. The purpose of this article was to (1) examine the relationship between self-chosen sexual orientation la-

Diane Powers, MA, is affiliated with the Fred Hutchinson Cancer Research Center, 1100 Fairview Ave., N. MP-900, Seattle, WA 98109.

Deborah J. Bowen, PhD, is now also affiliated with the Fred Hutchinson Cancer Research Center.

Jocelyn White, MD, is affiliated with Legacy Good Samaritan Medical Center, 1130 NW 22nd Ave., Suite 220, Portland, OR 97210.

Address correspondence to: Deborah J. Bowen, PhD, Fred Hutchinson Cancer Research Center, 1100 Fairview Ave. N., MP900, Seattle, WA 98109.

This research was supported by grants from the National Human Genome Institute, the National Cancer Institute, and the Office for Research on Women's Health (HG/CA 01190).

[Haworth co-indexing entry note]: "The Influence of Sexual Orientation on Health Behaviors in Women." Powers, Diane, Deborah J. Bowen, and Jocelyn White. Co-published simultaneously in *Journal of Prevention & Intervention in the Community* (The Haworth Press, Inc.) Vol. 22, No. 2, 2001, pp. 43-60; and: *Prevention Issues for Women's Health in the New Millennium* (ed: Wendee M. Wechsberg) The Haworth Press, Inc., 2001, pp. 43-60. Single or multiple copies of this article are available for a fee from The Haworth Document Delivery Service [1-800-342-9678, 9:00 a.m. - 5:00 p.m. (EST). E-mail address: getinfo@haworthpressinc.com].

© 2001 by The Haworth Press, Inc. All rights reserved.

43

bels and other sexual orientation measures and (2) compare the health related behaviors of women of diverse sexual orientations based on simple sexual orientation measures. The participants in this study were women aged 18 to 74 recruited via public announcements in mainstream and minority communities to participate in a randomized trial of breast cancer risk counseling strategies. Sexual orientation, relevant health behaviors and other outcomes related to breast cancer risk and screening were measured. No single measure of sexual behavior or desire appears to accurately measure lesbian sexual orientation. Lesbians were found to participate in mammography and Pap testing at significantly lower levels than bisexuals and heterosexuals. These data add to the growing body of knowledge on lesbian health and point to areas of community action and future research. *[Article copies available for a fee from The Haworth Document Delivery Service: 1-800-342-9678. E-mail address: <getinfo@haworth pressinc.com> Website: <http://www.HaworthPress.com> © 2000 by The Haworth Press, Inc. All rights reserved.]*

KEYWORDS. Lesbian health, sexual orientation, health behaviors, mammography, Pap testing

INTRODUCTION

The investigation of diverse sexual orientations and associated health outcomes is emerging as an important research area (Institute of Medicine, 1999). Sexual orientation may influence health behaviors, risk for disease, and health outcomes in at least two important ways. First, lesbians may have differential risk of negative health outcomes for specific diseases because of a different prevalence of risk factors for those diseases due to lower rates of early detection. One hypothesis is that lesbians may be at increased risk for breast cancer based on a confluence of risk factors more prevalent in lesbians (Haynes, 1994; Denenberg, 1995; Brownworth, 1993; Gallagher, 1997; Brandt, 1993). These risk factors include higher reported rates of nulliparity (Gage, 1994; Bradford, Ryan, & Rothblum, 1994) and alcohol consumption (Skinner & Otis, 1992; Skinner, 1994; McKirnan & Peterson, 1989) compared with heterosexual women. Second, lesbians may perform health screening behaviors at different rates than heterosexual women. Lesbians reported that they were half as likely as heterosexual women to get mammograms and to perform regular breast self-examination (Trippet & Bain, 1992; Deevy, 1990; Polena, Gillispie, Lederman, &

O'Hara, 1994), thereby losing the 25% survival benefit attributed to such screening. If lesbians have lower rates of early detection because of lower rates of performing screening behaviors, this could lead to higher mortality.

Another risk factor for negative health outcomes that may be important for lesbians is lack of access to appropriate health care services. Barriers to access may be both economical and cultural. Despite higher education levels, lesbians report lower average household incomes and are less likely than heterosexual women to have health insurance coverage (Bradford & Ryan, 1988; Bybee & Roeder, 1990). Lack of financial resources to support health might lead to difficulty in getting care. Lesbians who have health insurance and/or the economic means to purchase health care services may still have difficulty receiving appropriate care. Homophobia in health care providers has been well documented (Cochrane & Mays, 1988; Mathews, Booth, Turner, & Kessler, 1986; Randall, 1989), and lesbians report discriminatory experiences alter revealing their sexual orientation to their health care provider (Lehmann, Lehmann, & Kelly, 1998; Stevens & Hall, 1988; Warshofsky, 1992). Even lesbians with access to sensitive care may still experience difficulty receiving appropriate care from a health care provider who is uninformed about lesbian health issues. For example, some health care providers erroneously believe that lesbians do not need cervical cancer screening (Ferris, Batish, Wright, Cushing, & Scott, 1996). These differential health risks and behaviors may lead to poorer health outcomes for lesbians.

But because no population-based investigations that include sexual orientation as a variable have been published to date, it is unknown whether lesbians have poorer health outcomes than heterosexual women. One study compared health behaviors among lesbians and heterosexual women attending a lesbian clinic in San Francisco, but methodological problems severely limit the interpretability of that study (Roberts, Dibble, Scanlon, Paul, & Davis, 1998). Two of the biggest problems to date in lesbian health research have been lack of standardized measures of sexual orientation and sampling bias (Sell & Petrulio, 1996). Lesbians who are affiliated with the lesbian community are relatively easy to reach, but these lesbians may differ in important ways from those who are not active in the community. One solution would be to identify a sexual orientation measure or scale that is simple enough to be incorporated as a standard demographic variable in data collection instruments not focused on sexual behavior and that could be used in a broad variety of health investigations.

Such a measure needs to be both simple and accurate in identifying lesbians. Single-item self-label measures (e.g., *"What is your sexual orientation: heterosexual, homosexual, bisexual, other?"*) are succinct, but they rely on study subjects' identifying with a particular label. Laumann, Gagnon, Michael, and Michaels (1994) and Sell, Wells, and Wypi (1995) found substantial incongruity between sexual behavior, desire, and identity, suggesting that a single-item self-label may not be an accurate measure of sexual orientation. Measuring the gender of one's current partner is another option, but this method alone does not allow for identification of, for example, currently celibate lesbians. These shortcomings suggest the need for better measures of sexual orientation.

The recent report of the Institute of Medicine (1999) on lesbian health lists the identification of better methods of measuring sexual orientation as one of three research priorities. A second priority is the determination of differential health risks. The purpose of this article is to (1) examine the relationship between multiple measures of sexual orientation and (2) compare the health-related behaviors of women of diverse sexual orientations. We broadened our investigations to include several health-related measures because many of these measures have been related to health screenings in previous research.

METHODS

Overview

Women (829) were recruited to participate in a randomized trial of breast cancer risk counseling. The study sample included women from the greater Seattle area who had a family history of breast cancer and women from three minority communities (African American, Ashkenazi Jewish, and lesbian) who may or may not have had a family history of breast cancer. These communities were targeted for focused recruitment because of their potentially heightened perceptions of risk for breast cancer incidence or mortality. All potential participants were screened for eligibility. Eligible participants completed a baseline questionnaire and, if still eligible, were randomized to a counseling condition or a delayed counseling/control condition. Sexual orientation, various health behaviors, and other outcomes related to breast cancer risk and screening were measured at baseline and follow-up. The long-term outcomes for the counseling research were decreased anxiety about breast cancer and increased intentions to obtain appropriate breast cancer screening. This article will focus on baseline data for women from all four studies (mainstream and three minority communities).

Recruitment and Baseline Assessment

Women from the general community were recruited via local area broadcast and print media outlets and large company employee newsletters. Women (357) were recruited via mainstream methods, with an announcement in a daily Seattle newspaper yielding the most participants. Women from the three minority communities were recruited primarily from community organizations/events and mailing lists. The Jewish Federation of Seattle is the largest local Jewish organization. A mailing to their membership list yielded more participants than any other single source. Together with other recruitment methods, 220 Ashkenazi Jewish women joined the study. A small notice in one of Seattle's daily newspapers announcing a study for African American women and recruitment at local African American churches yielded a total of 103 participants. The Gay and Lesbian Employee Network (GLEN) is an umbrella organization of gay and lesbian employee groups in the Pacific Northwest and produced the highest yield from the lesbian community. Most of these groups are located at large employers in the Seattle area (Microsoft, Boeing, University of Washington, etc.). An e-mail message was sent to the GLEN contacts at these organizations and they were asked to disseminate it to their membership. Together with other strategies (e.g., announcement in local lesbian newspapers), 149 participants were recruited through the lesbian community methods.

In response to prompts from the various recruitment methods, women called the research center. Study staff completed a brief telephone survey to screen for eligibility. Eligibility criteria for the study included participants between ages 18 and 74 with no personal history of breast or ovarian cancer, residing within 60 miles of Seattle, having a family cancer pedigree not indicative of an inherited autosomal dominant predisposition to breast cancer, and indicating a willingness to complete surveys and participate in breast cancer risk counseling. Information on family history of cancer was collected via a self-report form. Participants were asked to identify the number of each type of first- or second-degree blood relative they have (e.g., *"How many sisters does your mother have?"*), whether the relative ever had cancer and, if so, the type, age of diagnosis, and whether or not the relative was still living. A family cancer pedigree was defined as indicative of an autosomal dominant predisposition to breast cancer if it met either of these criteria: (1) two or more first-degree or one first-degree and one second-degree relative with either breast cancer before age 50 or ovarian cancer at any age or (2) at least two paternal second-degree relatives with either breast cancer before age 50 or ovarian cancer at any age. These guidelines were adapted from those published by Kaiser Permanente (Kutner, Formanek, & Bergoffen, 1995) to represent women at genetic risk for breast cancer who should be considered for referral to a genetics clinic. Women meeting these guidelines were excluded from the breast cancer counseling trial because one of the conditions was a delayed counseling/control condition, which was not considered an appropriate option for them. Women recruited from the general community were required to have a family history of breast cancer. Women from the three minority communities were not, and about half the women in each of these samples reported a family history of breast cancer.

Eligible participants were mailed a packet containing a consent form and a self-administered baseline survey to complete and return to the research center in a provided postage-paid envelope. Women who did not return the baseline survey to the research center within two weeks were given a reminder call.

Assessments

Sexual orientation measures for all the study samples included self-label and gender of past sexual partner(s). The self-label item asked participants to choose from the list: heterosexual, lesbian/gay/homosexual, bisexual, transgendered, or other. Gender of past sexual partner(s) was adapted from a long-term study of women's health, the Women's Health Initiative (Matthews et al., 1997), which asked participants to report the gender of their adult sexual partner(s). Except those recruited via the lesbian community, this was the limit of sexual orientation measures. For women recruited via the lesbian community, the sexual orientation measures were expanded to include gender of current partner, first sexual partner, preferred partner, partner in sexual fantasies, partner in sexual dreams, persons for whom you feel erotic/sexual desire, and preferred life partner.

Demographic information was collected using simple single-item measures. Education level, race, income level, employment status, and marital/partner status were all assessed using standard categorical response choices. Age was measured in years.

Health behaviors were measured and included the frequency of participation in breast and cervical cancer screening, alcohol consumption, exercise activities, and cigarette use. Simple single-item measures were used. For example, for the questions "How often have you had mammograms in the past?" and "How often do you have Pap smears?", women responded using closed-ended categories.

Participants reported their weight in pounds and their height in feet and inches. These items were converted to metric equivalents and body mass index calculated (weight/height^2).

General anxiety and depression were measured using the Brief Symptom Inventory (Derogatis & Melisaratos, 1983). This instrument is a reliable, valid measure of emotional and psychiatric variables consisting of 49 items with five-point scales. Their responses were calculated into mean subscales, including anxiety and depression. Overall mental health was measured using the SF-36 (Ware, Snow, Kosinki, & Gandek, 1993), which is a multi-item, well validated, and widely used quality-of-life instrument that includes a mental health subscale. Cancer worry was measured with the Cancer Worry Scale (Lerman, Rimer, Trock, Balshem, & Engstrom, 1990). This widely used survey is a four-item scale with four-point response categories measuring the frequency of worry about breast cancer and its impact on functioning. The answers range from "Not at all or rarely" to "A lot." The minimal score is 4 and the maximum possible score is 16. The alpha coefficient for this questionnaire is approximately 0.7 in other research (Lerman & Schwartz, 1993).

Data were analyzed in several steps. All study samples were combined to form one large dataset. Participants in the combined study sample were divided by self-identified sexual orientation labels (lesbian, bisexual, heterosexual). Demographic variables among sexual orientation categories were examined. Next, the self-identified sexual orientation label was compared to (1) behavior and desire variables for lesbians and bisexual women in the lesbian study only and (2) behavior in the combined sample. Health behaviors and psychological variables among sexual orientation categories were calculated in the combined study sample, using ANOVA and chi-square tests where appropriate. Post hoc comparisons were conducted using a Tukey test, where appropriate. Finally, the frequencies of mammography and Pap screening were predicted using logistic regression (0 = below recommendations and 1 = at or above recommendations). Sexual orientation and demographic variables significantly related to sexual orientation as predictor variables were all entered simultaneously.

RESULTS

Table 1 shows the population characteristics for participants from the combined study group according to self-identified sexual orientation label. Cross tabulation of demographic variables revealed several significant differences. Ethnicity differed among sexual orientation categories significantly, likely because of the inclusion of women recruited from the African American community in the heterosexual category. Age, education, income, employment status, and marital status were also significantly different among study sexual orientation groups. There was no relationship found between family history of breast cancer or other reproductive risk factors for breast cancer and sexual orientation (data not shown).

Table 2 displays the data on sexual behavior and desire for participants recruited from the lesbian community who self-labeled as lesbian/gay and as bisexual. Cross tabulation of all sexual behavior and desire variables showed significant differences between lesbians and bisexuals, except for "first partner." Over half of both groups reported having a male as a first sexual partner. Of the women who used the label "lesbian," the majority reported having a past male partner. Only a slight majority (53%) of bisexuals recruited through the lesbian community reported that their current partners were only women, and 12% reported that their past partners were all women. Regarding desire, only 86% of self-identified lesbians reported that they strongly prefer women. Sixty-five percent of bisexuals recruited via the lesbian community reported that they prefer women to some degree, as compared with 29% with no preference and 6% who prefer men. Slightly less than half of the self-identified lesbians reported erotic/

TABLE 1. Population Characteristics

	Lesbians (%) (n = 152)	Bisexuals (%) (n = 30)	Heterosexuals (%) (n = 647)
Age[a]			
Under 40	46	50	36
40 or over	54	50	64
Ethnicity[a]			
White	93	97	79
Other	7	3	21
Education[a]			
4-Year College Graduate or Less	45	37	65
Professional Degree	55	63	35
Income[b]			
<$15,000	7	14	6
$15,000 - 29,999	20	21	13
$30,000 - 49,999	31	24	25
$50,000 - 69,999	17	21	21
≥ $70,000	24	21	35
Employed[a]			
Full Time	76	50	50
Part Time	13	27	25
Not Employed/Retired	11	23	26
Marital/Partner Status[a]			
Married/Living with a Partner	53	57	64
Single/Widowed/Separated/ Divorced	47	44	36

[a] $p < .01$
[b] $p < .05$

sexual desire for women only, though 86% preferred only women for life partners. Interestingly, 11% of lesbians prefer "mostly women" for a life partner, and 2% would consider a man for a life partner.

We performed a factor analysis of principal components with varimax rotation using four sexual orientation items from the sample of women recruited from the lesbian community: current partner, past partner, preferred partner gender, and gender in fantasy for life partner. The items loaded onto a single factor, accounting for 77% of the variance. We used the responses from the two highest-loading questions (with current woman partner loading 0.9 and preference for woman life partner loading 0.89) to classify the participants who endorsed the label "lesbian" and found that the responses to the two questions correctly classified 99% of the participants who endorsed the label of "lesbian."

Table 3 compares past sexual partners to reported self-label for the entire study sample. Cross tabulation of past sexual behavior with self-label was significant among sexual orientations, as expected.

TABLE 2. Sexual Orientation Identity, Behavior and Desire for Lesbians and Bisexuals

	Self-Label	
	Lesbian/Gay (%) (n = 132)	Bisexual (%) (n = 17)
	Behavior	
Current Partner[a]		
Only Women	87	53
Mostly Women	2	12
Both Men and Women	–	6
Only Men	–	6
Not Sexually Active	11	24
Past Partner(s)[b]		
Women Only	43	12
Men Only	2	6
Both	55	82
First Partner		
Female	41	18
Male	59	82
	Desire	
Preferred Partner Gender[a]		
Strongly Prefer Women	86	6
Prefer Women	14	59
No Preference	–	29
Prefer Men	–	6
Partner's Gender in Sexual Fantasies[a]		
Only Women	36	6
Mostly Women	33	12
Both Men and Women	27	82
Mostly Men	2	–
No Fantasies	2	–
Partner's Gender in Sexual Dreams[a]		
Only Women	21	–
Mostly Women	46	6
Men and Women	26	88
Mostly Men	2	–
Don't Have Sexual Dreams	6	6
Erotic/Sexual Desire[a]		
Only Women	49	6
Mostly Women	43	29
Men and Women	7	59
Mostly Men	–	6
No Desire	1	–
Preference for Life Partner[a]		
Only Women	86	12
Mostly Women	11	59
Women or Men	2	29

[a] $p < .01$
[b] $p < .05$

TABLE 3. Sexual Orientation Identity and Behavior for Entire Study Sample

	Self-Label		
	Lesbian (%) (n = 152)	Bisexual (%) (n = 30)	Heterosexual (%) (n = 641)
Behavior			
Past Partner(s)[a]			
Women Only	42	7	-
Men Only	3	20	98
Both	55	73	1
Never Had Sex	-	-	1

[a]$p < .01$

Virtually all heterosexual women reported men only for their past sexual partners, whereas lesbians and bisexuals reported a diversity of past sexual partners. In particular, over half of the lesbians and bisexuals reported past sex with both women and men.

Health behavior findings are included in Table 4. There were no differences in cigarette smoking, alcohol consumption, or moderate or strenuous exercise frequency among sexual orientations. For both breast and cervical cancer screening behaviors, the data were dichotomized based on the national recommendations for obtaining screening at least once every two years. Mammography behaviors were reported for women over age 40 in each category. Reporting of Pap smear data was not age-restricted because the general national recommendations specify only that all women 18 and over should participate in regular cervical cancer screening. Reported frequency of screening mammography was significant among sexual orientation categories. Visual inspection of the data in Table 4 shows that lesbians reported less frequent mammograms compared with both bisexuals and heterosexuals. Frequency of Pap smears followed the same pattern, in that lesbians reported a significantly lower frequency of obtaining Pap smears than did either bisexual women or heterosexual women (χ^2 = 45.0, p < .000). Emotional well-being findings from the baseline survey and body mass index results from the six-month follow-up survey are included in Table 5. Mental health subscores on the Quality-of-Life Scale were higher for heterosexual women, compared with lesbians or bisexual women. No other emotional or physical variables showed differences among sexual orientation categories.

TABLE 4. Health Behaviors and Psychological Variables for Entire Study Sample

	Lesbians (%) (n = 132)	Bisexuals (%) (n = 30)	Heterosexuals (%) (n = 647)
Currently Smoke	7	10	7
Alcohol Use			
Rarely/Never	28	40	25
1-3 Times/Month	38	37	43
1-2 Times/Week	17	13	16
3-4 Times/Week	9	3	8
Nearly Every Day or More	7	7	7
Mild Exercise			
Rarely/Never	5	13	7
Few Times a Month	19	7	18
1-2 Times/Week	28	13	26
3-5 Times/Week	30	40	29
About Every Day	18	7	20
Strenuous Exercise			
Rarely/Never	38	37	33
Few Times a Month	15	10	17
1-2 Times/Week	20	30	18
3-5 Times/Week	24	20	26
Every Day	2	3	5
Pap Test Frequency[a]			
Less Than Every 2 Years	20	10	9
Every 2 Years or More	80	90	91
Mammography Frequency[a]	(n = 81)	(n = 15)	(n = 414)
Less than Every 2 Years	26	13	12
Every 2 Years or More	74	87	88

[a] $p < .01$

TABLE 5. Psychological Variables and Body Mass Index for Entire Study Sample

	Lesbians (SD) (n = 132)	Bisexuals (SD) (n = 30)	Heterosexuals (SD) (n = 647)
QOL: Mental Health[a]	72 (15)	72 (15)	76 (14)
BSI: Anxiety	0.46 (0.46)	0.46 (0.41)	0.40 (0.46)
BSI: Depression	0.48 (0.57)	0.49 (0.52)	0.42 (0.52)
Cancer Worry	5.95 (1.8)	6.37 (2.1)	6.04 (1.8)
Body Mass Index	(n = 124)	(n = 23)	(n = 353)
	27.1 (5.9)	26.9 (8.0)	25.9 (6.0)

[a] $p < .05$

Table 6 shows the results of logistic regression predicting frequency of mammography and Pap screening using sexual orientation and selected demographic variables. As seen in this table, sexual orientation category was a significant predictor of frequency for both types of screening, when other demographic variables were included in the equation. In particular, reporting a heterosexual label improved chances of obtaining mammography and Pap smear significantly. The other significant predictor of mammography was higher income, and the other significant predictor of Pap smear was being employed.

DISCUSSION

Differences among the sexual orientation categories in key demographic variables provide information for formulating hypotheses about potential health differences in these populations. Lesbians reported higher educational levels yet lower household incomes than did heterosexual women and bisexual women. Given the consistent relationship between economic status and health, this might indicate one pathway for lesbians' potential health decrements relative to women involved with men.

One significant demographic difference was in marital status

TABLE 6. Predicting Screening Frequency Using Sexual Orientation and Selected Demographic Variables

	Recommended Mammography		Recommended Pap Smear	
	Odds Ratio	Confidence Interval	Odds Ratio	Confidence Interval
Sexual Orientation				
Lesbian* vs. Bisexual	0.53	0.34, 8.6	0.84	0.65, 8.3
Lesbian* vs. Heterosexual	1.7	1.12, 3.12[b]	1.3	2.0, 5.7[a]
Caucasian* vs. Other	0.40	0.83, 2.7	0.35	0.8, 2.6
Four-Year Degree				
or Below* vs.	0.95	0.56, 1.59	0.37	0.9, 2.3
Higher				
Employed* vs. Not	0.56	0.30, 1.03	0.76	1.3, 3.6[a]
Partnered* vs. Not	1.18	0.66, 2.09	0.43	0.89, 2.6
Income Below 50K* vs. Higher	1.4	1.11, 1.80[a]	0.90	0.72, 1.12

[a] p < .01
[b] p < .05
* Referent Group

among lesbians, bisexuals, and heterosexuals. The higher prevalence of lesbians who are not living with a partner may be due to cultural differences that have their root in the prohibition of homosexual marriage. Lesbian culture has produced alternatives to the traditional model of heterosexual marriage (Kurdek, 1988). As a result, lesbians may have more sexual partners over the course of their lifetime and be less likely to live with their partner than their heterosexual counterparts. More research is needed in this area.

The development of simple, accurate measures of sexual orientation and their inclusion in a broad spectrum of health studies is necessary to broaden our understanding of the health risks and behaviors of lesbians. Our data suggest that no single measure of sexual behavior or desire is adequate as a substitute for self-label. However, self-label is also limited in its ability to accurately measure sexual orientation. Past sexual behavior is inadequate because of the large number of self-identified lesbians who have had male partners in the past. Measuring current sexual behavior provides no information about women who are currently celibate. Desire did not function as an adequate substitute for self-label because a surprisingly high number of self-identified lesbians did not report that they "strongly prefer" a woman for a sexual or life partner and less than half report erotic/sexual desire for women only.

It may be possible to construct a subset of behavior, desire, and self-label variables to simply and accurately measure sexual orientation. One question about self-identified sexual orientation captures currently celibate individuals as well as those who identify with the self-label. Current sexual behavior and desired gender of sexual partner could be used to capture individuals who do not identify with the self-label. Additional research, especially with a more population-based sample, is needed to determine if such a combination of these three questions can be used to measure sexual orientation in a broad variety of health investigations.

Our findings support the need for additional research into health behavior differences between lesbians and non-lesbians. The finding that lesbians are significantly less likely than non-lesbians to participate in routine mammography and Pap screening needs further study on larger samples with more population-based recruitment strategies.

This study measured mammography and Pap testing rates by self-report. So, for lesbians who report less-frequent mammograms and

Pap smears, it is unclear whether their health care providers did not recommend them, whether the women did not go to get screened of their own accord, or whether they failed to report mammograms and Pap tests that they did obtain. There is no plausible reason why sexual orientation should influence self-reporting. While there is no evidence to suggest that health care providers recommend mammograms less frequently for their lesbian patients, there is some evidence (Ferris et al., 1996) to suggest that health care providers do not believe that lesbians need cervical cancer screening. This could stem from the erroneous belief that most lesbians have had only female sexual partners and so are not at risk for transmission of HPV (human papillomavirus), though there is preliminary data to suggest that female-to-female transmission of HPV is also possible (O'Hanlan & Crum, 1996). It is also possible that lesbians may fail to seek Pap screening because they believe themselves to be at lower risk for cervical cancer than bisexual and heterosexual women (Price, Easton, Telljohann, & Wallace, 1996). Another factor that may influence rates of participation in both mammography and Pap testing is that lesbians may see their health care provider less frequently than bisexual and heterosexual women and thereby have fewer opportunities to receive recommendations for breast and cervical screening (White & Dull, 1997). There were no differences between lesbians and non-lesbians in cancer worry, so a heightened fear of cancer is not a likely explanation for less frequent mammography.

The only psychological variable that differed among sexual orientation categories was mental health. Lesbians and bisexual women may have lower mental health levels than heterosexuals because they may be less identified with the dominant, mainstream community than with the lesbian community. They may experience lower mental health levels either because they attempt to conceal their sexual orientation or because they are exposed to discrimination if they do not conceal it.

This study has several limitations that constrain the generalizeability of the findings to a broad group. First, the recruitment method was based on self-selection. Women of all sexual orientations volunteered for a study conducted by health researchers. It can be difficult for researchers to find and recruit lesbians into health studies. One of the strengths of this study is that researchers were able to recruit a cohort of lesbians who were demographically similar to women recruited from the general population. However, both samples were self-selected for interest in breast cancer risk information, giving some strength to the presumption that the differences within the sample across sexual orientation categories are real. Our findings point to the need for further study of differences in health behaviors between lesbians and non-lesbians and potential reasons for these differences. A second limitation is the relatively small sample size for some variables, a factor that produces small cells in some comparisons and prohibits us from controlling for many different potential confounders in multivariate analyses. These findings do, however, provide support for the idea that in large samples of women one can ask successfully about sexual orientation without reducing response in other areas of the survey for heterosexual women. This information should help other investigators to include simple measures of sexual orientation in large ongoing studies of women's health.

REFERENCES

Bradford, J., & Ryan, C. (1988). *The national lesbian health care survey* (Final Report). Washington, DC: National Lesbian and Gay Health Foundation.

Bradford, J., Ryan, C., & Rothblum, E. (1994). National lesbian health care survey: Implications for mental health care. *Journal of Consulting and Clinical Psychology, 62*, 28-242.

Brandt, K. (1993). Lesbians at risk. *Deneuve, Sept./Oct.*, 34-37.

Brownworth, V.A. (1993). The other epidemic: Lesbians and breast cancer. *Out, Feb/March.*

Bybee, D., & Roeder, V. (1990). *Michigan lesbian health survey: Results relevant to AIDS. A report to the Michigan Organization for Human Rights and the Michigan Department of Public Health.* Lansing, MI: Department of Health and Human Services.

Cochrane, S., & Mays, V.M. (1988). Disclosure of sexual preference to physicians by black lesbian and bisexual women. *Western Journal of Medicine, 149*, 616-619.

Deevy, S. (1990). Older lesbian women: An invisible minority. *Journal of Gerontological Nursing, 16*, 35-39.

Denenberg, R. (1995). Report on lesbian health. *Women's Health Issues, 5*, 81-91.

Derogatis, L.R., & Melisaratos, N. (1983). The brief symptom inventory: An introductory report. *Psychological Medicine, 13*, 595-605.

Ferris, D., Batish, S., Wright, T., Cushing, C., & Scott, E. (1996). A neglected lesbian health concern: Cervical neoplasia. *Journal of Family Practice, 43*, 581-584.

Gage, S. (1994). *Preliminary findings: National lesbian and bi-women's health survey.* Presented at the National Lesbian and Gay Health Conference, New York, NY.

Gallagher, J. (1997). Lesbians and breast cancer. *The Advocate, 30*, 20-27.

Haynes, S. (1994). Risk of breast cancer among lesbians. Presented at the Cancer and Cancer Risk Among Lesbians Interactive Conference, Seattle, WA.

Institute of Medicine. (1999). *Lesbian health: Current assessment and directions for the future.* Committee on Lesbian Health Research Priorities. Washington, DC: National Academy Press.

Kurdek, L.A. (1988). Relationship quality of gay and lesbian cohabiting couples. *Journal of Homosexuality, 15,* 93-118.

Kutner, S., Formanek, R., & Bergoffen, J. (1995). *Clinical practice guidelines for breast cancer screening.* Kaiser Permanente Northern California Region, Breast Cancer Task Force, *June.*

Laumann, E.O., Gagnon, J.H, Michael, R.T., & Michaels, S. (1994). *The social organization of sexuality: Sexual practices in the United States.* Chicago, IL: University of Chicago Press.

Lehmann, J.B., Lehmann, C.U., & Kelly, P.J. (1998). Development and health care needs of lesbians. *Journal of Women's Health, 7,* 379-387.

Lerman, C., Rimer, B., Trock, B., Balshem, A., & Engstrom, P.F. (1990). Factors associated with repeat adherence to breast cancer screening. *Preventive Medicine, 19,* 279-290.

Lerman, C., & Schwartz, M. (1993). Adherence and psychological adjustment among women at high risk for breast cancer. *Breast Cancer Research and Treatment, 28,* 145-155.

Mathews, W.C., Booth, M.W., Turner, J.D., & Kessler, L. (1986). Physicians' attitudes toward homosexuality: Survey of a California County Medical Society. *Western Journal of Medicine, 144,* 106-110.

Matthews, K., Shumaker, S., Bowen, D.J., Langer, R.D., Hunt, J.R., Kaplan, R., Klesges, R., & Ritenbaugh, C. (1997). Women's health initiative: Why now? What is it? What's new? *American Psychologist, 52,* 101-116.

McKirnan, D.J., & Peterson, P. (1989). Alcohol and drug use among homosexual men and women: Epidemiology and population characteristics. *Addictive Behaviors, 14,* 545-563.

O'Hanlan, K.A., & Crum, C.P. (1996). Human papillomavirus-associated cervical intraepithelial neoplasia following lesbian sex. *Obstetrics & Gynecology, 88,* 702-709.

Polena, B., Gillispie, B., Lederman, D., & O'Hara, T. (1994). *Lesbian health care survey.* Denver, CO: Presbyterian/St. Luke's Medical Center.

Price, J.H., Easton, A.N., Telljohann, S.K., & Wallace, P.B. (1996). Perception of cervical cancer and Pap smear screening behavior by women's sexual orientation. *Journal of Community Health, 21,* 89-105.

Randall, C. (1989). Lesbian phobia among BN educators: A survey. *Journal of Nursing Education, 28,* 302-306.

Roberts, S., Dibble, S., Scanlon, J., Paul, S., & Davis, H. (1998). Difference in risk factors for breast cancer: Lesbian and heterosexual women. *Journal of Gay and Lesbian Medical Association, 2,* 93-101.

Sell, R., & Petrulio, C. (1996). Sampling homosexuals, bisexuals, gays, and lesbians for public health research: A review of the literature from 1990-1992. *Journal of Homosexuality, 30,* 31-47.

Sell, R., Wells, J., & Wypi, D. (1995). The prevalence of homosexual behavior and attraction in the United States, the United Kingdom and France: Results of national population-based samples. *Archives of Sexual Behavior, 24*, 235-48.

Skinner, W., & Otis, M. (1992). Drug use among lesbians and gay people: Findings, research, design, insights, and policy issues from the Trilogy Project. In *Proceedings of the Research Symposium on Alcohol and Other Drug Problem Prevention Among Lesbians and Gay Men* (pp. 34-60). Sacramento, CA: Evaluation, Management and Training Group, Inc.

Skinner, W. (1994). The prevalence and demographic predictors of illicit and licit drug use among lesbians and gay men. *American Journal of Public Health, 84*, 1307-1310.

Stevens, P., & Hall, J. (1988). Stigma health beliefs and experiences with healthcare in lesbian women. *Journal of Nursing School, 20*, 69-73.

Trippet, S., & Bain, J. (1992). Reasons American lesbians fail to seek traditional health care. *Health Care for Women International, 13*, 145-153.

Ware, J., Snow, K., Kosinki, M., & Gandek, B. (1993). *SF36 health survey: Manual and interpretation guide*. Boston: Nimrod Press.

Warshofsky, L. (1992). *Lesbian health needs assessment*. Los Angeles, CA: Gay and Lesbian Community Services Center.

White, J.C., & Dull, V.T. (1997). Health risk factors and health seeking behavior in lesbians. *Journal of Women's Health, 6*, 103-112.

Reduction of Co-Occurring Distress and HIV Risk Behaviors Among Women Substance Abusers

Susan Reif
Wendee M. Wechsberg
Research Triangle Institute

Michael L. Dennis
Chestnut Health Systems

SUMMARY. Women who abuse alcohol and drugs may have a number of co-occurring distress issues, such as depression, traumatic stress, and violence, that impede their ability to make changes in the behaviors that place them at risk for contracting HIV. The objective of this article is to evaluate the influence of participating in an enhanced HIV risk-reduction project on reducing women's co-occurring distress. Study partici-

Susan Reif, PhD, and Wendee M. Wechsberg, PhD, are affiliated with the Research Triangle Institute, Research Triangle Park, NC 27709.

Michael L. Dennis, PhD, is affiliated with Chestnut Health Systems, 720 West Chestnut, Bloomington, IL 61701.

Address correspondence to: Wendee M. Wechsberg, PhD, Senior Research Psychologist, Research Triangle Institute, 3040 Cornwallis Road, Research Triangle Park, NC 27709.

This work was supported by the National Institute on Drug Abuse (Contract No. 1-U01-DA-08007-01-AI). The interpretations and conclusions do not represent the position of NIDA or the Department of Health and Human Services.

The authors would like to thank Sallie West for her assistance in preparing the manuscript.

[Haworth co-indexing entry note]: "Reduction of Co-Occuring Distress and HIV Risk Behaviors Among Women Substance Abusers." Reif, Susan, Wendee M. Wechsberg, and Michael L. Dennis. Co-published simultaneously in *Journal of Prevention & Intervention in the Community* (The Haworth Press, Inc.) Vol. 22, No. 2, 2001, pp. 61-80; and: *Prevention Issues for Women's Health in the New Millennium* (ed: Wendee M. Wechsberg) The Haworth Press, Inc., 2001, pp. 61-80. Single or multiple copies of this article are available for a fee from The Haworth Document Delivery Service [1-800-342-9678, 9:00 a.m. - 5:00 p.m. (EST). E-mail address: getinfo@haworthpressinc.com].

© 2001 by The Haworth Press, Inc. All rights reserved.

61

pants were 206 predominantly African-American women who participated in the North Carolina CoOperative (NC CoOp) Study that
provided AIDS outreach to crack and injection drug users. The women
participated in a two-session standard risk-reduction intervention and
were then randomly assigned to either receive no further intervention or
to participate in an additional three-session-enhanced intervention. The
enhanced intervention was designed to work with individual participants in the context of their specific needs and co-occurring distress issues. Co-occurring distress, including depression, anxiety, traumatic
stress, victimization, aggression, and physical health, was measured at
intake and at 3 months after the intervention. The reduction in co-occurring distress was much more substantial for participants receiving the
enhanced intervention. In addition, the difference in reduction of co-occurring distress between the standard and enhanced intervention groups
was the greatest for women who reported the highest levels of baseline
co-occurring distress. These findings suggest that a longer, more personalized intervention may be expected to produce greater positive
changes in the lives of women who exhibit a high degree of distress.
Reduction in co-occurring distress can improve women's quality-of-life
and may enhance their ability to subsequently reduce their HIV risk behavior. *[Article copies available for a fee from The Haworth Document Delivery
Service: 1-800-342-9678. E-mail address: <getinfo@haworthpressinc.com> Website: <http://www.HaworthPress.com> © 2001 by The Haworth Press, Inc. All
rights reserved.]*

KEYWORDS. Women, HIV risk, substance abuse, mental distress

INTRODUCTION

Gender differences in HIV risk have been well documented in
recent years. For example, the rate of HIV infection has increased
more rapidly among women than men. In 1992, women accounted for
13.8% of persons living with AIDS, and by 1998 this proportion had
risen to 23% (CDC, 1999). Women are more likely to be infected
through heterosexual contact or injection drug use, whereas the leading source of transmission for men is male-to-male sexual contact.

It has also been well established that all women are not equally at
risk. Most HIV cases are found among young, minority, indigent
women who use crack cocaine and trade sex for crack, other drugs, or
money (Holmberg, 1996). While African Americans comprise about
12% of the population, they account for 56% of all AIDS cases among
women, and AIDS is the leading cause of death among African-American women (Anderson, Kochanek, & Murphy, 1997).

Despite the general recognition that women's risk is different than men's, the environmental or clinical basis of that difference has not been fully explored in the literature. However, some studies have found that, in addition to drug abuse, women often have contextual issues or co-occurring problems that may influence their participation in HIV risk behavior as well as their ability to reduce HIV risk. For example, clinical studies of women entering drug treatment show that women report lower self-concepts and more emotional symptoms–including depression and anxiety–than men (Blume, 1986; De Leon & Jainchill, 1986; Griffin, Weiss, Mirin, & Lange, 1989; Wallen, 1992; Wechsberg, Craddock, & Hubbard, 1998a) and that they are significantly more likely than men to show evidence of affective and psychotic disorders (Calsyn, Fleming, Wells, & Saxon, 1996). Studies have also indicated that women report more physical problems than men (Anderson, 1990), more childhood sexual abuse (Boyd, Blow, & Orgain, 1993; Murphy, Stevens, McGrath, Wexler, & Reardon, 1998; Rohsenow, Corbett, & Devine, 1988; Titus, White, Dennis, & Scott, in press; Wechsberg et al., 1998a; Wallen, 1992; Murphy et al., 1998), and more physical abuse (Ladwig & Andersen, 1989; Wechsberg et al., 1998a) than their male counterparts. In addition, women have been found to demonstrate more psychosexual disorders and anorexia nervosa (Fornari, Kent, Kabo, & Goodman, 1994; Ross, Glaser, & Stiasny, 1988). Furthermore, for women of low socioeconomic status, AIDS is only one of many life problems and is often rated as being less serious than unemployment, lack of child care, and crime victimization (Stevens & Bogart, 1999; Sterk, 1999; Kalichman, Hunter, & Kelly, 1992).

Clearly, these studies demonstrate a greater prevalence of emotional distress and other issues that occur in the context of women's lives, which may influence their decisions about engaging in high-risk activities and negatively impact their ability to reduce their HIV risk behavior. Higher levels of emotional distress may reduce women's capacity to evaluate their ability to change behavior or protect themselves. For example, the sense of hopelessness and despair that often is characteristic of depression may interfere with the adoption of safer behaviors to prevent HIV infection (Orr, Celentano, Santelli, & Burwell, 1994). Additional sequelae of emotional distress that may influence HIV risk behavior and behavior change include poor impulse control, self-destructive behavior, and lack of assertiveness and effective communication skills. Assertiveness and communication skills are often necessary to negotiate the use of protective behavior with sexual or needle-sharing partners.

A number of studies examined the relationship between emotional distress and risk behavior and found that substance abusers with higher levels of emotional distress demonstrate significantly greater HIV risk behavior (Camacho, Brown, & Simpson, 1996; Bell, 1996; McCusker, Goldstein, Bigelow, & Zorn, 1995). Reduction of this co-occurring distress has been hypothesized to result in a subsequent decline in HIV risk behavior. Several studies (Nyamathi, Bennett, & Leake, 1995; McCusker et al., 1995) provide some support for an association between reduction in distress and reduction in HIV risk behavior after participation in an HIV prevention intervention. These studies found that persons who demonstrated greater reduction of distress were more likely to demonstrate higher levels of HIV risk reduction (Nyamathi et al., 1995; McCusker et al., 1995).

Many HIV prevention programs have focused solely on providing HIV education and behavior skills training and have not addressed the co-occurring issues and conditions that are prominent in women's lives. Given the complexity of women's problems, it is not surprising that these HIV prevention programs often have limited success in reducing the risk behaviors. When women bring to the prevention program a range of problems, the program's ability to help them reduce risk may be hampered by the varied co-occurring conditions that act as barriers. Furthermore, to the extent that these HIV risk behaviors are intimately related to the social context of the women's lives and to their physical and mental health, a comprehensive approach to interventions for risk reduction may be indicated to effect real change among women at high risk for contracting HIV. Woody, Metzger, Navaline, McLellan, and O'Brien (1997) summarized the results of studies that explored the benefit of adding a focus on psychiatric issues to addiction-focused drug treatment. These studies provided evidence that substance-abusing patients with high-severity co-occurring problems made few gains when given drug counseling alone, whereas those who received additional supportive-expressive or cognitive-behavioral psychotherapy made significant gains. While HIV preventions are not designed to provide drug treatment, they are structured to focus on reducing drug use, entering drug treatment, and reducing sexual risk. It would seem to follow that HIV prevention interventions, like drug treatment, would benefit from adding a focus on psychiatric problems and other co-occurring distress issues that may act as barriers to the goals of HIV prevention intervention (Wechsberg et al., 2000).

The purpose of this study was to explore the extent of distress in the lives of women at high risk for contracting HIV and to examine the question of whether a personalized intervention directed at addressing contextual and co-occurring distress issues can be more successful in reducing women's co-occurring distress than a standard two-session HIV risk-reduction intervention.

METHODS

Data Source. Data for this study were collected as part of the North Carolina CoOperative Agreement for AIDS Community-Based Outreach, Intervention, and Research (NC CoOp) (Wechsberg et al., 2000). The NC CoOp program was one of 23 sites in the U.S. and abroad funded by NIDA that targeted out-of-treatment injection drug users and crack users for HIV risk reduction and research. The objectives of the NIDA project included establishing a system for monitoring the nature and extent of drug use and HIV-related risk behaviors in out-of-treatment drug users and assessing the efficacy of established interventions in reducing risk behaviors among out-of-treatment drug users (Wechsberg, Dennis, & Stevens, 1998b). Wechsberg et al. (2000) found that women in both the standard and enhanced intervention groups significantly reduced their alcohol and crack use, trading-sex behavior, and unprotected sex acts. However, women in the enhanced intervention demonstrated significantly greater reductions in alcohol use and overall substance abuse than women who only participated in the brief standardized intervention.

Participants. To be included in the study, an individual had to (a) provide informed consent, (b) be over 18 years old, (c) have been out of treatment for at least 30 days, (d) report injection or crack drug use in the past 30 days, and (e) have either visible needle tracks or a positive urine test for opiates or cocaine. The participants in the NC CoOp randomized study were recruited from a metropolitan county in North Carolina between February 1995 and August 1998.

Participants were blocked by gender, whether they were injection drug users, and whether they had multiple sexual partners and then, within blocks, were randomly assigned at a 2:3 ratio to either the standard or standard plus enhanced interventions. Blocking allows us to treat the women as being in a separate experiment, as we have done here. We used a 2:3 ratio because it was assumed that not all of the women would be willing to come back for the three additional sessions in the enhanced intervention. Participation was voluntary and conducted under the supervision of RTI's institutional review board for human subjects. Participants were given an incentive of $35 for each interview completed.

Study Subsample. The subsample of the NC CoOp sample used for this study consisted of 206 predominantly African-American substance-abusing women, primarily crack users, participating in the NC CoOp who had been randomized at a 2:3 ratio to either the standard (n = 84) or standard plus enhanced (n = 122) interventions. Of the total of 206 women who were initially randomized to the standard and enhanced interventions, 33 (16%) were not available for follow-up. Attrition analysis, using chi-square tests and t-tests, was performed to determine whether key characteristics were significantly different for participants who were lost to follow-up and participants who completed the study. The women who did not complete the study were younger, were more likely to inject drugs, and reported less alcohol use than women who completed the study. A similar analysis was performed to detect differences in the characteristics of women randomized to the standard and enhanced interventions. Only race was found to differ significantly between the groups, as the standard intervention had 12 white participants, and the enhanced intervention had 7.

Instruments. Data were collected by self-report using NIDA's Risk Behavior Assessment (RBA), the standard instrument used at all Co-Operative Agreement sites. The RBA is an 80-item questionnaire that collects information on demographic characteristics and sexual and drug risk behaviors. The RBA has been found to be a reliable and valid research tool for use with persons who use illicit drugs (Weatherby et al., 1994; Dowling-Guyer et al., 1994). Data were also obtained from a second, site-specific instrument, the NC CoOp's Trailer II, a 64-item questionnaire designed to assess contextual issues in the respondent's life, including physical health, mental health, and victimization. The Trailer II assessment consisted of existing and tested scales, including the Physical Health Distress Scale (Dennis, 1999; Titus et al., in press), an adapted version of the DATAR Depression

Scale (Simpson, 1992), the DATAR Anxiety Index (Simpson, 1992), the General Conflict Tactic Scale (Strauss, 1990; Dennis, 1999), the General Victimization Scale (Dennis, 1999; Titus et al., in press), and an adapted version of the Traumatic Stress Disorder Index (Kulka et al., 1990; Dennis, 1999). The Physical Health Distress Scale contained items such as self-reported health status, activity limitations, and physical pain. The victimization scale focused on emotional, physical, and sexual abuse in the previous 90 days, while the conflict scale, which measures aggressive behavior, consisted of questions about verbal or physical violence toward another person. The scales demonstrated acceptable internal consistency reliability in the NC CoOp sample with Cronbach's Alpha scores of .7 and higher (Wechsberg et al., 1998b). The RBA was administered at intake, and the Trailer II was administered at a second session, normally within 2 weeks of intake. Follow-up data were collected at 3 months with the Risk Behavior Follow-up Assessment (RBFA), an instrument similar to the RBA, and with the Trailer II again.

Standard Intervention. All NC CoOp participants received the revised version of NIDA's standard intervention (Wechsberg et al., 1997; Wechsberg et al., 1998c). This consisted of two sessions of HIV education and counseling supported by a standard set of cue cards that addressed injecting risk, risk from crack use, and sexual risk. Participants were asked to role-play and rehearse condom use and needle cleaning, and they were offered referrals to other service providers as necessary. HIV antibody testing and posttest counseling were also included for patients who consented to be tested.

Enhanced Intervention. About 60% of the participants completing the standard intervention were then randomized into the enhanced intervention, which consisted of three additional sessions. At the first session, participants were given a personalized risk assessment showing where their reported behaviors placed them with respect to the behaviors of the study population. Using that information, they worked with the counselor to develop a personal plan for risk reduction, which included addressing co-occurring distress and other contextual factors. The next two sessions were interactive and devoted to problem-solving, communication skills, and rejecting drug offers and risky sex. Case managers attempted to contact enhanced intervention participants on a weekly basis to follow up on referrals made for treatment and/or other community services and to encourage participants to continue working on their risk-reduction goals. Because of the higher intensity of the enhanced intervention and the fact that it focused on issues specific to each individual, participants in the enhanced intervention were hypothesized to demonstrate greater reduction in HIV risk behaviors as well as co-occurring distress issues, such as emotional distress.

Statistical Methods. Descriptive statistics, including means and proportions, were calculated to provide information about demographic characteristics and co-occurring distress issues in the sample of women. Every participant was assigned a score on each of the six co-occurring distress scales, which included depression, anxiety, traumatic stress, aggression, victimization, and physical health, by adding their responses to the individual items in the scale. For some individual scale items, the response categories were reversed so that a higher score would indicate a higher level of that specific measure of co-occurring distress. Baseline scores from the six co-occurring distress scales were added for each individual to create a co-occurring distress score. The co-occurring distress score demonstrated adequate internal consistency reliability with a Cronbach's Alpha score of .75. The women were then divided into high and low co-occurring distress groups by the median co-occurring distress score in order to evaluate differences in co-occurring stress reduction by the level of baseline co-occurring distress. Demographic characteristics and substance use patterns were compared between the high and low co-occurring groups by using t-tests and chi-square tests.

To examine the changes between pre-intervention and post-intervention for the co-occurring distress scales, we conducted t-tests to determine statistical significance and then focused on the effect sizes to measure practical significance. This is important because of both the limited sample size and concerns for a Type II error. Because we hypothesize both mean and variance effects, we based the error term on the standard group only (see Dennis, Lennox, & Foss, 1997 for a further discussion on this issue). To measure pre- to posttest changes, we calculated:

T-Test   t = (mean post-intervention–mean pre-intervention)/(standard error pre)

Effect Sized   d = (mean post-mean pre)/(standard deviation pre)

To determine whether the enhanced intervention was significantly better at reducing co-occurring distress than the standard intervention, we calculated the difference score (post-pre) for each individual and then calculated the T-Tests and effect sizes as:

Relative T-Test   t = (mean difference enhanced–mean difference standard)/(standard error difference standard)

Relative Effect Size d = (mean difference enhanced–mean difference standard)/(standard deviation difference standard)

Following common recommendations set forth elsewhere (Cohen, 1988; Dennis et al., 1997), we consider effect sizes of greater than 0.2 to be meaningful, while effects in the range of +.2 to − .2 should be considered to be little or no change for practical purposes. All effect sizes have been scaled so that positive (up) is bad and negative (down) is good (i.e., reduced drug use, sexual risk, co-occurring distress, etc.). An intention-to-treat approach was used to assess the changes in co-occurring distress from pre- to post-intervention and between standard and enhanced groups in order to preserve the integrity of the randomized design. This means that we have analyzed women based on the condition to which they were assigned regardless of whether they actually went to the additional treatment. Because of the high attrition, we also calculated the outcomes in two ways as recommended by Stanton and Shadish (1997). First, the 33 women without follow-up data were assumed to have made no improvement from baseline to follow-up, so their change scores on the distress scales were set to zero, and their follow-up scores on the distress measures were set to their pre-intervention score. Second, the analysis was performed without the missing women (de facto, assuming an average outcome). Results between the two approaches demonstrated were nearly identical, so we have only reported the former here.

RESULTS

Description of the Sample. Women in the NC CoOp study demonstrated relatively high levels of co-occurring distress. For example, a majority of women reported at least sometimes experiencing most of the symptoms of depression and anxiety. Just over half of the women indicated that they often or almost always feel sad or depressed. When asked whether they felt interested in life, 27% of the women reported only sometimes feeling interested in life, and 20% reported rarely or never having this feeling. In addition, over a third of the women reported at least sometimes experiencing nearly all of the 12 symptoms of traumatic stress. Ten percent of the women responded "almost always" to the item "When I think of some of the things I have done in the past, I wish I were dead." Aggressive acts were common in the sample, as 70% had insulted or sworn at someone else in the past 90 days, and nearly half reported having pushed, grabbed, or shoved someone in the previous 90 days. Victimization was also very prevalent in the sample of drug-using women. Two-thirds of the women reported that they had been physically, sexually, or emotionally abused in the 90 days prior to the baseline interview. In addition, health problems were common in the sample, as 70% of the women reported at least one negative physical health symptom or activity limitation, and close to 50% reported two or more negative health symptoms or activity limitations.

Tables 1 and 2 show selected demographic characteristics and co-occurring distress scores of the total sample and by distress group. The high distress group, those with co-occurring distress scores greater than the median "total distress" score, tended to be younger and reported a higher level of criminal activity. Unemployment was common in the high and low distress groups, as more than half of the women in both groups reported not being employed. The high distress group was significantly more likely to have been in drug treatment either in the previous 90 days or ever. In addition, the high distress group was significantly more likely to be homeless, with nearly 40% being homeless compared to 12% of the low distress group. In both the high and low distress groups, nearly all of the women (greater than 95%) reported crack use in the 30 days prior to the interview. The prevalence of injecting was low for both groups, but a substantially larger proportion of the high distress group reported both injecting and crack use. The high distress group was also significantly more likely to trade sex for drugs or money. As expected, because of the randomized study design, the proportions of people in the standard and en-

TABLE 1. Selected Baseline Characteristics for the Total Sample and by Co-Occurring Distress Group[a]

	Proportion of Low Distress N = 103	Proportion of High Distress Group N = 102	Total Sample
Age			
18-25	.08	.10	.09
26-35	.46	.54	.48
36-45	.35	.32	.34
46 and over	.13	.06	.09
Less than high school diploma	.37	.42	.40
Married	.21	.23	.22
Unemployed	.66	.68	.67
Homeless	.13	.34**	.24
Intervention received			
Standard	.38	.43	.40
Enhanced	.62	.57	.60
Ever been in drug treatment	.45	.62**	.53
Mental health treatment in previous 90 days	.03	.08	.05
Sexual activity			
Celibate	.11	.13	.12
Heterosexual	.88	.85	.86
Lesbian	.01	.02	.02
Baseline risk behavior (all behaviors are for the 30 days before RBA)			
Had unprotected sex	.72	.75	.73
IDU only	.02	.06	.04
Crack only	.78	.65	.72
Both IDU and crack	.19	.29	.24
Traded sex for drugs or money	.18	.40**	.29

* $p < .05$ for tests of the difference between high and low co-occurring distress groups.
**$p < .01$.

[a]Total distress score is based on the sum of depression, anxiety, traumatic stress, victimization, aggression, and health symptom counts; high vs. low group based on a median split of the sample.

hanced groups who reported high levels of distress were virtually equal.

Reduction in Co-Occurring Distress. For the entire sample of women that participated in the NC CoOp randomized experiment, significant reductions from pre- to post-intervention were noted for depression, anxiety, aggression, and overall co-occurring distress; marginally significant declines were detected for traumatic stress, victimization, and health (see Table 3 for the pre- to post-intervention reduction in co-occurring distress measures). Analyzing the sample of women by treatment assignment (standard or enhanced) reveals striking differences in

TABLE 2. Baseline Co-Occurring Distress Scores for the Total Sample and by Co-Occurring Distress Group[a]

Baseline Co-Occurring Distress	High Co-Occurring Distress Group N = 86	Low Co-Occurring Distress Group N = 86	Total Sample
Depression	16.67**	9.74	13.19
Anxiety	16.34**	6.94	11.62
Traumatic Stress	25.81**	9.63	17.68
Aggression	5.60**	2.37	3.97
Victimization	4.44**	2.18	3.31
Physical Health	6.38**	4.10	5.23
Total Distress*	75.24**	34.68	55.00

* $p < .05$ for tests of the difference between high and low co-occurring groups.
** $p < .01$.

[a]Total distress score is based on the sum of depression, anxiety, traumatic stress, victimization, aggression, and health symptom counts; high vs. low group based on a median split of the sample.

reduction of co-occurring distress between treatment groups. Among women in the standard intervention, there were no major pre- to post-intervention reductions on the co-occurring distress measures for depression, traumatic stress, anxiety, physical health, and victimization. In contrast, the women in the enhanced intervention reported statistically significant reductions in all six co-occurring distress scales. The reduction in overall distress for the enhanced group was significantly larger than the overall distress reduction for the standard group (see Table 4 for comparison of pre- to post-intervention reductions between the standard and enhanced intervention groups). Although differences in reduction of the specific co-occurring distress scales between standard and enhanced participants were only identified to reach statistical significance for anxiety, the effect sizes for the differences between standard and enhanced participants for depression, physical health, and victimization reduction were all .20 or higher.

Comparison of Change in Co-Occurring Distress by High and Low Co-Occurring Distress Group. Stratification of the sample by baseline distress levels provides more information about the differences between standard and enhanced intervention groups with respect to reduction of co-occurring distress from pre- to post-intervention. When comparing the high and low distress groups, created by dividing the distress scores at the median, only the high distress group showed substantial improvement for all six of the co-occurring distress scales

TABLE 3. Change in Co-Occurring Distress from Pre- to Post-Intervention

Index	T-test Comparing Baseline to Follow-up			Effect Size of Change from Baseline to Follow-up		
	Standard	Enhanced	Total	Standard	Enhanced	Total
Depression	−1.28	−3.39**	−3.44**	−.14	−.31	−.24
Anxiety	.47	−3.23**	−2.25*	.05	−.29	−.16
Traumatic Stress	−.64	−1.81	−1.81	−.07	−.16	−.13
Victimization	−.01	−2.36*	−1.82	−.01	−.21	−.13
Aggression	−1.74	−1.91	−2.59*	−.18	−.17	−.18
Physical Health	−.24	−2.20*	−1.94	−.03	−.20	−.14
Total Distress[a]	−.64	−3.09**	−2.8*	−.07	−.28	−.20

* $p < .05$.
** $p < .01$.

[a]Total distress score is based on the sum of depression, anxiety, traumatic stress, victimization, aggression, and health symptom counts.

TABLE 4. Comparison of the Changes in Co-Occurring Distress from Pre- to Post-Intervention Between the Standard and Enhanced Intervention Groups

	T-test (Standard vs. Enhanced)	Effect Size (Standard vs. Enhanced)
Depression	1.76	.20
Anxiety	3.60**	.40
Traumatic Stress	1.05	.16
Victimization	1.82	.20
Aggression	−.23	−.02
Physical Health	1.89	.21
Total Distress[a]	2.68*	.29

* $p < .05$.
** $p < .01$.

[a]Total distress score is based on the sum of depression, anxiety, traumatic stress, victimization, aggression, and health symptom counts.

(see Table 5 for t-tests comparing pre- and post-intervention change in co-occurring distress for high and low co-occurring distress groups). With the exception of aggression, the decrease in co-occurring distress from baseline to follow-up for women with higher baseline distress was only statistically significant for enhanced intervention participants. For aggression, women with high levels of distress in both the standard and enhanced interventions showed substantial improvement. The effect sizes for reduction of co-occurring distress were also larger for high distress women in the enhanced group than similar women in the standard group. In addition, t-tests that compared distress reduction between standard and enhanced intervention participants indicated the difference in co-occurring distress reduction for high distress women in the enhanced intervention to be significantly greater than the distress reduction for similar women in the standard intervention for depression, anxiety, physical distress, and overall co-occurring distress (see Table 6 for a comparison of the t-tests and effect sizes between the standard and enhanced interventions for the high and low co-occurring groups).

In contrast with women experiencing higher levels of distress at baseline, women with lower levels of baseline co-occurring distress in either the standard or enhanced group demonstrated no substantial reduction in victimization, physical health distress, anxiety, traumatic stress, or aggression. Furthermore, women in the lower distress group who participated in the standard intervention actually demonstrated an increase in anxiety. For depression, women in the low co-occurring distress group in the enhanced intervention demonstrated some decrease in their depressive symptoms (effect size of .2), whereas similar women in the standard intervention showed little change in depression. In the low distress groups, no significant changes in either traumatic stress or aggression were detected.

TABLE 5. Change in Co-Occurring Distress from Pre- to Post-Intervention Stratified by Low and High Distress Groups[a]

	Standard Intervention				Enhanced Intervention			
	T-test Comparing Baseline to Follow-up		Effect Size of Change from Baseline to Follow-up		T-test Comparing Baseline to Follow-up		Effect Size of Change from Baseline to Follow-up	
	Low Distress N = 34	High Distress n = 37	Low Distress	High Distress	Low Distress N = 52	High Distress N = 49	Low Distress	High Distress
Depression	−.31	−1.84	−.05	−.28	−1.94	−4.19**	−.24	−.55
Anxiety	2.37*	−.59	.38	−.09	−.18	−6.18**	−.02	−.81
Traumatic Stress	1.32	−1.70	.21	−.26	−.86	−2.98**	−.11	−.39
Aggression	.39	−2.66*	.06	−.40	.06	−2.88**	.01	−.38
Physical Health	.95	−.72	.15	−.11	.29	−2.98**	.04	−.39
Victimization	.46	−.49	.07	−.07	−1.29	−2.53*	−.16	−.33
Total Distress	1.76	−2.45*	.28	−.37	−1.32	−5.90**	−.17	−.78

* p < .05.
** p < .01.

[a]Total distress score is based on the sum of depression, anxiety, traumatic stress, victimization, aggression, and health symptom counts; high vs. low group based on a median split of the sample.

TABLE 6. Comparison of Pre- and Post-Intervention Changes Between Standard and Enhanced Interventions for the Low and High Co-Occurring Distress Groups[a]

	Low Co-Occurring Distress (n = 86) Standard vs. Enhanced		High Co-Occurring Distress (n = 86) Standard vs. Enhanced	
	Relative t-Test	Relative Effect Size	Relative t-Test	Relative Effect Size
Depression	.72	.10	2.29*	.34
Anxiety	1.52	.24	4.21**	.63
Traumatic Stress Disorder	1.56	.25	.42	.06
Aggression	.40	.06	−.36	−.05
Physical Health	.94	.15	2.41*	.36
Victimization	1.16	.19	1.51	.23
Total Distress	1.80	.30	2.38*	.36

* $p < .05$.
** $p < .01$.

[a]Total distress score is based on the sum of depression, anxiety, traumatic stress, victimization, aggression, and health symptom counts; high vs. low group based on a median split of the sample.

DISCUSSION

The fact that women's risk for HIV infection differs from men's in important ways poses difficult challenges for interventions. Specifically, women's vulnerability to various forms of co-occurring distress suggests that HIV risk-reduction interventions that focus only on drug and sexual behaviors may not be sufficient to effect real change in women's lives. Co-occurring distress issues, such as emotional distress and abuse, may inhibit women's ability to focus and feel comfortable making the changes necessary to reduce HIV risk. The NC CoOp enhanced intervention, which included the development of a personal risk reduction plan, referrals to community agencies that could assist with substance abuse and specific co-occurring distress issues, the setting of specific and concrete goals, and follow-up reminders of goals, represented an attempt to involve the whole person in the risk-reduction effort. The hypothesis behind this more holistic approach was that, by considering each woman in the context of her situation and the specific issues that contribute to her risk, the intervention would be more successful in reducing co-occurring distress and HIV risk behaviors.

Study results for women who participated in the NC CoOp randomized HIV prevention experiment provide support for the hypothesis that women with co-occurring distress may benefit from an intervention that focuses on some of their individual needs and concerns. Women who were assigned to the enhanced intervention reported greater reduction in overall co-occurring distress than women assigned to the standard intervention. When the women were divided into high and low distress groups by the median distress score, there were clear distinctions in reduction of co-occurring distress from pre- to post-intervention between the high and low distress groups. The high distress group showed more improvement than the low distress group, and those in the high distress group who received the enhanced intervention demonstrated significantly greater improvement than similar women who only participated in the standard intervention. These findings suggest that a longer, more personalized intervention may be expected to produce greater positive changes in women who exhibit a high degree of distress. Reduction of distress can improve women's quality of life and may make it easier for them to focus on reduction of behaviors that place them at risk for contracting HIV and other sexually transmitted diseases. Furthermore, the extra costs associated with the time committed to work individually with participants were found to be offset by the additional reduction in drug use associated with participation in the enhanced intervention (Zarkin, Lindrooth, Demiralp, & Wechsberg, in press).

The results of this study must be taken in the context of its limitations. Without a true control group that received no prevention intervention, determining the extent that the self-reported changes in each group resulted from the standard intervention is not possible, although both interventions did appear to produce positive outcomes. However, the randomized design for comparing behavior change between participants in the standard and enhanced interventions offered much greater protection against threats to validity such as a general trend for decrease in risk behavior and the influence of other community interventions. The relatively small sample size for this study, n = 206, may also have influenced study results due to a lack of power to detect statistically significant differences between study groups. However, we were able to at least partially address the issue of small sample size by including evaluation of effect sizes. In addition, because men were also involved in the NC CoOp study, the structure of the intervention was not exclusively focused on the needs and concerns of women. Ideally, an intervention to reduce women's co-occurring distress and sexual and drug use behavior would be designed to have an in-depth focus on even more contextual issues, such as housing, employment, social support, and sexual relationships, that are integral to the lives of women participating in the intervention.

Although it is unreasonable to expect any intervention to solve all the problems in these women's lives, the results of this study suggest that women exhibiting co-occurring distress may benefit most from an intervention that deals with some of the sources of this distress through counseling and skills-building. However, as the intervention was not exclusively woman-focused and relatively high levels of distress and risk persisted despite the declines that followed intervention participation, further study is necessary to determine whether an intervention specifically addressing women's co-occurring distress issues can be more effective in reducing HIV risk behaviors than one addressing drug and sexual risk alone. Longer and more personalized interventions that address co-occurring and contextual issues in women's lives may be more cost-effective, in the long term, than shorter interventions addressing HIV risk behaviors alone.

Additional study is also warranted to assess whether reduction of co-occurring distress results in greater reduction of HIV risk behaviors over time. Because baseline and follow-up measures of HIV risk and distress were taken simultaneously in this study, it was not possible to determine whether reduction in co-occurring distress resulted in subsequent reduction of risk behavior. Women whose co-occurring distress issues predated their substance abuse and who use substances to cope with this distress may require assistance to reduce their underlying distress before making lasting changes in substance use and HIV risk. In contrast, women whose distress emerged as a result of substance abuse may experience a decrease in co-occurring distress if they are able to reduce their use of substances. A longitudinal study of women at high risk for HIV is necessary to examine the role of reduction of distress in influencing the risk behavior of women at high risk of contracting HIV and other sexually transmitted diseases.

REFERENCES

Anderson, E. (1990). *Streetwise: Race, class and change in an urban community.* Chicago, IL: University of Chicago Press.

Anderson, R.N., Kochanek, K.D., & Murphy, S.L. (1997). *Report of final mortality statistics, 1995. Monthly vital statistics report, 45, Table 7.* Hyattsville, MD: National Center for Health Statistics.

Bell, D. (1996). The effects of psychosocial domains in AIDS risk behavior. *Drugs and Society, 9*, 37-55.

Blume, S.B. (1986). Women and alcohol: A review. *Journal of the American Medical Association, 256*, 1467-1470.

Boyd, C.J., Blow, F., & Orgain, L.S. (1993). Gender differences among African-American substance abusers. *Journal of Psychoactive Drugs, 25*, 301-305.

Calsyn, D.A., Fleming, C., Wells, E.A., & Saxon, A.J. (1996). Personality disorder subtypes among opiate addicts in methadone maintenance. *Journal of Addictive Disorders, 10*, 3-8.

Camacho, L.M., Brown, B.S., & Simpson, D.D. (1996). Psychological dysfunction and HIV/AIDS risk behavior. *Journal of Acquired Immune Deficiency Syndrome Human Retrovirol, 11*, 198-202.

Centers for Disease Control and Prevention (CDC). (1999). *HIV/AIDS among U.S. women: Minority and young women at continuing risk*, Atlanta, GA: Centers for Disease Control Publications.

Cohen, J. (1988). *Statistical power analysis for the behavioral sciences*. Hillsdale, NJ: Lawrence Erlbaum Associates.

De Leon, G., & Jainchill, N. (1986). Circumstances, motivation, readiness, and suitability as correlates of treatment tenure. *Journal of Psychoactive Drugs, 18*, 203-208.

Dennis, M.L. (1999). Global Appraisal of Individual Needs (GAIN): Administration guide for the GAIN and related measures. [On Line]. Bloomington, IL: Chestnut Health Systems. Available: http://www.chestnut.org/li/gain/gadm1299.pdf.

Dennis, M.L., Lennox, R.I., & Foss, M. (1997). Practical power analysis for substance abuse health services research. In K.J. Bryant, M. Windle, & S.G. West (Eds.), *The science of prevention: Methodological advances from alcohol and substance abuse research* (pp. 367-405). Washington, DC: American Psychological Association.

Dowling-Guyer, S., Johnson, M.E., Fisher, D.G., Needle, R., Watters, J., Anderson, M., Williams, M., Kotranski, L., Booth, R., Rhodes, F., Weatherby, N., Estrada, A.L., Fleming, D., Deren, S., & Tortu, S. (1994). Reliability of drug users self-reported HIV risk behaviors and validity of self-reported recent drug use. *Assessment, 1*, 383-392.

Fornari, V., Kent, J., Kabo, L., & Goodman, B. (1994). Anorexia nervosa: Thirty-something. *Journal of Substance Abuse Treatment, 11*, 45-54.

Griffin, M.L., Weiss, R.D., Mirin, S.M., & Lange, V. (1989). A comparison of male and female cocaine abusers. *Archives of General Psychiatry, 46*, 122-126.

Holmberg, S.D. (1996). The estimated prevalence and incidence of HIV in 96 large U.S. metropolitan areas. *The American Journal of Public Health, 86*, 642-654.

Kalichman, H.C., Hunter, T.C., & Kelly, T.C. (1992). Perceptions of AIDS susceptibility among minority and non-minority women at risk for HIV infection. *Journal of Consulting and Clinical Psychology, 60*, 725-732.

Kulka, R.A., Schlenger, W.E., Fairbank, J.A., Hough, R.L., Jordan, B.K., Marmar, C., & Weiss, D. (1990). *Trauma and the Vietnam war generation: Report of findings from the National Veterans Readjustment Study*. New York, NY: Brunner Mazel.

Ladwig, G.B., & Andersen, M.D. (1989). Substance abuse in women: Relationship between chemical dependency of women and past reports of physical and/or sexual abuse. *International Journal of the Addictions, 24*, 739-754.

McCusker, J., Goldstein, R., Bigelow, C., & Zorn, M. (1995). Psychiatric status and HIV risk reduction among residential drug abuse treatment clients. *Addiction, 90*, 1377-1387.

Murphy, B.S., Stevens, S.J., McGrath, R, Wexler, H.K., & Reardon, D. (1998). Women and violence: A different look. *Drugs and Society, 13(1/2)*, 131-144.

Nyamathi, A.M., Bennett, C., & Leake, B. (1995). Predictors of maintained high-risk behaviors among impoverished women. *Public Health Reports, 110*, 600-606.

Orr, S.T., Celentano, D.D., Santelli, J., & Burwell, L. (1994). Depressive symptoms and risk factors for HIV acquisition among black women attending urban health centers in Baltimore. *AIDS Education and Prevention, 6*, 230-236.

Rohsenow, D., Corbett, R., & Devine, D. (1988). Molested as children: A hidden contribution to substance abuse? *Journal of Substance Abuse Treatment, 5*, 13-18.

Ross, H.E., Glaser, F.B., & Stiasny, S. (1988). Sex differences in the prevalence of psychiatric disorders in patients with alcohol and drug problems. *British Journal of Addiction, 83*, 1179-1192.

Simpson, D.D. (1992). *TCU/DATAR forms manual*. Fort Worth, TX: Texas Christian University.

Stanton, M.D., & Shadish, W. (1997). Outcome, attrition, and family-couples treatment for drug abuse: A meta-analysis and review of the controlled, comparative studies. *Psychological Bulletin, 122*, 170-191.

Sterk, C.E. (1999). *Fast lives: Women who use crack cocaine*. Philadelphia: Temple University Press.

Stevens, S.J., & Bogart, J.G. (1999). Reducing HIV risk behavior of drug involved women: Medical, social, economic and legal constraints. In W.N. Elwood (Ed.), *Power in the blood: AIDS, politics and communication*, Mahweh, NJ: Lawrence Erlbaum Associates, 107-120.

Strauss, M.A. (1990). Conflict Tactic Scales. In M.A. Straus & R.I. Gelles (Eds.), *Physical violence in American families: Risk factors and adaptations to violence in 8,145 families*. Durham, NH: University of New Hampshire.

Titus, J.C., White, W., Dennis, M.L., & Scott, C. (in press). Gender differences in the severity and patterns of victimization among adolescents treated for substance abuse: Intake status and outcomes. Problems of Drug Dependence 2000: Proceedings of the 62nd Annual Scientific Meeting: The college of Problems on Drug Dependence, Inc., *NIDA Research Monograph*. Rockville, MD: National Institute on Drug Abuse.

Wallen, J. (1992). A comparison of male and female clients in substance abuse treatment. *Journal of Substance Abuse Treatment, 9*, 243-248.

Weatherby, N.L., Needle, R., Cesari, H., Booth, R., McCoy, C., Watter, J., Williams, M., & Chitwood, D. (1994). Validity of self-reported drug use among injection drug users and crack cocaine users recruited through street outreach. In M.L. Dennis & W.M. Wechsberg (Eds.), Special Issue: Evaluating Drug Abuse Interventions. *Evaluation and Program Planning, 17*, 347-355.

Wechsberg, W.M., MacDonald, B.R., Dennis, M.L., Inciardi, J.A., Surratt, H.L.,

Leukefeld, C.G., Farabee, D., Cottler, L.B., Compton, W.M., Hoffman, J., Klein, H., Desmond, D., & Zule, B. (1997). *The standard intervention for reduction in HIV risk behavior: Protocol changes suggested by the continuing HIV/AIDS epidemic.* Bloomington, IL: Lighthouse Institute. Available online: http://www.chestnut.org/li/publications.

Wechsberg, W.M., Craddock, S.G., & Hubbard, R.L. (1998a). How are women who enter substance abuse treatment different than men? A gender comparison from the Drug Abuse Treatment Outcome Study (DATOS). *Drugs and Society, 13,* 99-117.

Wechsberg, W.M., Dennis, M.L., & Stevens, S.J. (1998b). Cluster analysis of HIV outcomes among substance-abusing women. *American Journal of Drug and Alcohol Abuse, 24,* 239-257.

Wechsberg, W.M., Desmond, D., Inciardi, J.A., Leukefeld, C.G., Cottler, L.B., & Hoffman, J. (1998c). HIV prevention protocols: Adaptation to evolving trends in drug use. *Journal of Psychoactive Drugs, 30,* 291-298.

Wechsberg, W., Dennis, M., McDermeit, M., Perritt, R., Middlesteadt, R., & Reif, S. (2000). A comparison by gender of the main effects of a brief intervention with a longer personalized skills building approach. *1999 CPDD Proceedings: NIDA Research Monograph.*

Woody, G.E., Metzger, D., Navaline, H., McLellan, T., & O'Brien, C.P. (1997). Psychiatric symptoms, risky behavior, and HIV infection. *NIDA Research Monograph 172,* 156-170.

Zarkin, G.A., Lindrooth, R.C., Demiralp, B., & Wechsberg, W.M. (In Press). The cost and cost-effectiveness of an enhanced intervention for out-of treatment substance abusers. *Health Services Research.*

Perception of Health Status and Participation in Present and Future Health Promotion Behaviors Among African-American Women

Catherine M. Waters
University of California–San Francisco

Rita Times
City and County of San Francisco Department of Public Health

Agnes Rolle Morton
Oceanview, Merced Heights, and Ingleside Community Action Organization

Mildred Crear
City and County of San Francisco Department of Public Health

Mercy Wey
University of California–San Francisco

Catherine M. Waters, PhD, RN, and Mercy Wey, MSN, RN, are affiliated with the University of California–San Francisco, Department of Community Health Systems, School of Nursing. Rita Times, MSN, PHN, RN, and Mildred Crear, MSN, MA, PHN, RN, are affiliated with City & County of San Francisco Department of Public Health, California Children Services. Agnes Rolle Morton, MPH, MSN, PHN, RN, is affiliated with Oceanview, Merced Heights, and Ingleside Community Action Organization.

Address correspondence to: Catherine M. Waters, PhD, RN, Assistant Professor, Department of Community Health Systems, University of California–San Francisco, School of Nursing, 2 Kirkham Street, San Francisco, CA 94143-0608 (E-mail: catherine.waters@nursing.ucsf.edu).

[Haworth co-indexing entry note]: "Perception of Health Status and Participation in Present and Future Health Promotion Behaviors Among African-American Women." Waters, Catherine M. et al. Co-published simultaneously in *Journal of Prevention & Intervention in the Community* (The Haworth Press, Inc.) Vol. 22, No. 2, 2001, pp. 81-96; and: *Prevention Issues for Women's Health in the New Millennium* (ed: Wendee M. Wechsberg) The Haworth Press, Inc., 2001, pp. 81-96. Single or multiple copies of this article are available for a fee from The Haworth Document Delivery Service [1-800-342-9678, 9:00 a.m. - 5:00 p.m. (EST). E-mail address: getinfo@haworthpressinc.com].

© 2001 by The Haworth Press, Inc. All rights reserved.

SUMMARY. African-American women have a twofold prevalence of diabetes, hypertension, and stroke and nearly a threefold higher risk of overall mortality compared to Caucasian women. Many of these potentially preventable health conditions are related to lifestyle. The purpose of this small, cross-sectional, descriptive survey study was to describe the perceived health status, current health-promotion behaviors, and interest in participating in future health-promotion activities among African-American women. We then sought to determine if there was an association between perceived health status and current health-promotion behaviors, and between perceived health status and interest in participating in future health-promotion activities. We administered a modified version of the Behavioral Risk Factor Questionnaire (BRFQ) by mail or telephone to a convenience sample of 53 African-American women living in the San Francisco Bay area. In general, the fairly healthy women reported being physically inactive, eating primarily a low-fat diet, not smoking cigarettes or drinking, and coping fairly well with stress, but not eating the daily recommended five servings of fruits and vegetables. Findings revealed perceived health status was not associated with current health-promotion behaviors or interests in participating in future health-promotion activities. A majority of the women, however, were interested in participating in future health-promotion activities, such as a women's health program, nutrition improvement, and moderate physical activity, indicating potential opportunities for health-promotion interventions that engage African-American women in healthier lifestyles. To help an individual make a future change, such as one's health-promotion practices, health-promotion interventionists must understand the individual's present behavior in the context of that culture. *[Article copies available for a fee from The Haworth Document Delivery Service: 1-800-342-9678. E-mail address: <getinfo@haworthpressinc.com> Website: <http://www.HaworthPress.com> © 2001 by The Haworth Press, Inc. All rights reserved.]*

KEYWORDS. Health promotion, health status, women, African-American

BACKGROUND

African-American women have a twofold prevalence of diabetes, hypertension, and stroke and nearly a threefold higher risk of overall mortality compared to Caucasian women (American Heart Association, 1999). These health conditions, many of which are preventable and related to lifestyle factors, account for almost two-thirds of all United States medical expenditures and nearly three-quarters of all deaths (McGinnis & Foege, 1993). By changing individuals' negative lifestyle behaviors, health-promotion interventions can potentially improve longevity and quality of life, reduce the aggregate risk profile, and reduce health care costs. To design effective health-promotion interventions, there is a need to understand different groups' perceptions of health, their current health-promotion behaviors, and their readiness to engage in health-promotion practices, if necessary. The challenge is to understand health behaviors in the context of that "culture," which profoundly influences beliefs and behaviors. The concept of health has subjective meaning. Thus, what constitutes health, and what are considered appropriate methods of preventing and resolving health issues, might be determined culturally, socially, economically, environmentally, and/or politically.

During the late 1970s and early 1980s, three large community cardiovascular disease intervention studies were conducted to evaluate the effectiveness of comprehensive, community-wide health education on reducing the risks associated with cardiovascular disease, i.e., high dietary fat, hypertension, cigarette smoking, obesity, and sedentary lifestyle. The studies involved 12 cities, six of which received a 5- to 8-year multifactorial risk reduction program, in three distinct geographic regions of the United States. These studies consisted of the Stanford Five-City Project in California, the Minnesota Heart Health Program in the Minneapolis-St. Paul metropolitan areas, and the Pawtucket Heart Health Program in Rhode Island (Winkleby, Feldman, & Murray, 1997). These studies produced a wealth of knowledge about health behaviors, and many of the short-term targeted interventions within the larger studies were found effective. Long-term presumed effectiveness, however, was not seen. The recommendation was that more attention must be paid to finding ways to reach people who have resisted previous programs and messages, or subgroups that these studies were unable to reach. All three studies consisted predominantly of Caucasian, non-Hispanic participants (83% to 97%, $n = 5,792$), aged 25 to 64 years, with almost equal numbers of men and women. The principal ethnic minority group was Hispanic (6% to 10%). African-Americans represented 0.1% to 2.7% of the three combined samples. There is an overwhelming need to target, assess, and develop focused health-promotion interventions for women, ethnic minorities, older persons, and low socioeconomic persons, who continue to bear a disproportionate burden of morbidity and mortality (Krieger, Rowley, Herman, Avery, & Phillips, 1993; Nickens, 1995; Palank, 1991).

There are considerable gaps and conflicting findings in the knowledge of women's health, especially the health of African-American women (Eliason, 1999; Gary, Campbell, & Serlin, 1996; Landrine & Klonoff, 1997; Pinn, 1996; Rosenberg, Adams-Campbell, & Palmer, 1995). There have been limited studies that document the lack of participation in health-promotion behaviors among African-American women (Ahijevych & Bernhard, 1994; Felton, Parsons, Misener, & Oldaker, 1997; McCleary-Jones, 1996). There has been scant documentation that perceived health status might influence a woman's participation in healthy lifestyle behaviors (Calnan & Johnson, 1985), including ethnic-minority women (Martin & Panicucci, 1996; Sanders-Phillips, 1996). Furthermore, information is limited concerning the determinant of perceived health status on current health-promotion behaviors as it relates to a person's readiness for positive healthy behavior changes. Personal lifestyles may not be as simplistic as the informed or uninformed choices that people make everyday that affect their health. To change behavior, health-promotion opportunities, cultural interpretations, and group-specific attitudes need to be further explored.

While we have some insight about various groups of people's present health-promotion patterns, we are much less advanced in our knowledge of their readiness to change and their future interests in engaging in health promotion so that they can change unhealthy behaviors and enjoy the protective health benefits of living a healthier lifestyle. Self-assessment of health behaviors and readiness to change negative health behaviors among various subgroups of people is essential preliminary work that is necessary to facilitate measuring longitudinally sensitivity to changes in behaviors that result from health-promotion interventions. Thus, the purpose of this small, cross-sectional, descriptive survey study was to describe the perceived health status, current health-promotion behaviors, and interests in participating in future health-promotion activities among African-American women. We then sought to determine if there was an association between perceived health status and current health-promotion behaviors, and between perceived health status and interest in participating in future health-promotion activities.

THE THEORY OF PLANNED BEHAVIOR
AND THE TRANSTHEORETICAL MODEL
OF BEHAVIOR CHANGE

This study was contextually guided by the Theory of Planned Behavior's construct of behavioral intention (Ajzen, 1985) and the Transtheoretical Model of Behavior Change's construct of stages of change or level of preparedness to change (Prochaska & Velicer, 1997). According to the Theory of Planned Behavior, intention is postulated to be the primary determinant of behaviors under personal control. There is a strong focus on the relation between attitudes and behavior. Perceptions of beliefs of significant others about behavior are also hypothesized to be influential. Behavior is a result of a specific intention, determined by attitude toward the behavior and the subjective norm regarding that behavior. The Transtheoretical Model of Behavior Change acknowledges factors that hinder or promote the adoption and maintenance of positive health behaviors and brings into focus internal and external factors that influence individuals in their decision to make behavior changes. These internal and external factors often determine an individual's level of preparedness to change–precontemplation, contemplation, preparation, action, and maintenance–which influences self-efficacy and determines the gains (pros) and losses (cons) of changing behavior.

In this study, we were interested in African-American women's rating of their health status and whether the value rating of their health status was associated with their current health-promotion behaviors and their interest in participating in future health-promotion activities. We were particularly interested in women who were at the "preparation" stage of change: they intend to take action in the immediate future, measured as within the next month. We assumed that individual motivational factors determined the likelihood of the women engaging in a specific health-promotion behavior. We wanted to know if the women would be interested in participating in 15 specific health-promotion activities in the immediate future. These women would be ready for health-promotion interventions, especially since intentions are posited to be immediate antecedents to behavior. We believed that the women's current health-promotion practices were a function of their perceived health status, and that their perceived health status would determine their intent to engage in future health-promotion activities. For example, we hypothesized that women who rated their health as "excellent" or "poor" would have an attitude that health-promotion activities were unnecessary. In contrast, women who perceived their health as "very good," "good," or "fair" would have more interest in health-promotion activities.

METHODS

Design

A cross-sectional, descriptive survey design was employed to assess perceived health status, current health-promotion behaviors, and interests in participating in future health-promotion activities among African-American women. Future was defined as the individual intends to take action within a month. Data gathering was conducted in predominantly African-American communities throughout the San Francisco Bay area. The study was approved by the University of California, San Francisco, Committee on Human Research. Participant selection criteria were noninstitutionalized women who self-identified as African American, who were at least 18 years old, and who spoke and understood English.

Measure

Behavioral Risk Factor Questionnaire (BRFQ). A modified version of the BRFQ (Siegel, Frazier, Mariolis, Brackbill, & Smith, 1993) was used to survey a cross-section of African-American women about their perceived health status and current participation in four health-related lifestyle behaviors–physical activity, daily intake of fruits and vegetables, tobacco use, and alcohol intake. We added two questions regarding dietary fat and stress/coping. The BRFQ is a comprehensive measurement that includes questions from other widely known valid and reliable health population surveys, such as the RAND Health Survey, National Health Interview Survey, and the National Health and Nutrition Examination Survey (Siegel et al., 1993). The BRFQ collects data about modifiable health behaviors for chronic diseases and other leading causes of death, and sociodemographic characteristics. In the sociodemographic section, we added questions regarding family and personal health history of diabetes mellitus, cardiovascular disease, stroke, hypertension, cholesterol, and cancer. The BRFQ is designed to gather information from adults on actual health behaviors. The BRFQ is a structured, fixed-choice survey composed mostly of "yes/no" and "how often" responses. Its psychometric properties, including reliability and validity, have been documented (Bowlin et al., 1993; Bowlin, Morrill, Nafziger, Lewis, & Pearson, 1996; Brownson, Jackson-Thompson, Wilkerson, & Kiani, 1994; Giles, Croft, Keenan, Lane, & Wheeler, 1995), and there is support for its use in research involving ethnic minorities (Stein, Lederman, & Shea, 1993) and women (Stein, Lederman, & Shea, 1996). Reliability coefficients are generally above $r = .70$.

In addition, a question about the women's interest in participating in health-promotion activities within the next month was included in the survey. There were 15 health-promotion activities to which to respond. The response options were "yes" or "no." The list of activities was derived from focus group discussions with African-American women who lived in the study's targeted communities. The activities included a women's health program, nutrition improvement, health self-care, comprehensive health/fitness evaluation, stress management, weight management, walking, cancer risk reduction, aerobics with music, cholesterol reduction, heart risk reduction, blood pressure control, alcohol/drug reduction, jogging, and smoking cessation.

Procedure

A variety of nonrandom, convenience sampling and recruitment approaches were used, including network and snowball-sampling techniques. With ethnic-minority samples, these techniques typically yield a more representative sample and higher participation rates (Blumenthal, Sung, Coates, Williams, & Liff, 1995). Ethnic-minority participants generally recruit others whom they know and trust. The caveat is that these sampling methods present participant selection bias. Participants were invited through community liaisons, actively involved in predominantly African-American neighborhoods, churches and organizations, flyers, invitation letters, word-of-mouth, and presentations at community events and social gatherings, including health fairs, Easter egg hunts, and barber and beauty shops. Interested persons were able to contact the researcher by telephone using the number that both appeared on the printed materials and was announced at the various presentations, meetings, social gatherings, and forums.

Sixty interested African-American women who contacted the researcher and met sample selection criteria received a study description and assurance of confidentiality. Seven (12%) women did not complete the survey, yielding a final sample size of 53. Surveys were assigned a three-digit identification number. Participants were given the option to complete the BRFQ by mail ($n = 51$, 96%), telephone ($n = 2$, 4%), or face-to-face ($n = 0$, 0%). The primary researcher and one trained interviewer were responsible for data collection, monitoring, and tracking.

Surveys were distributed to interested participants who agreed voluntarily to participate in the study. The mailed packet contained the BRFQ, an addressed stamped envelope to return the survey, and an information sheet describing the study and the woman's rights as a research study participant. Follow-up reminders were not conducted. Telephone interviews were scheduled at a time convenient to the participant. A $25 remuneration was given to participants for completing the survey.

Data Analysis. Summary descriptive statistics were computed on the women's (a) sociodemographic characteristics, (b) perceived health status, (c) six currently practiced health behaviors (physical activity, dietary fat, fruits and vegetables, alcohol, tobacco, and stress/coping), and (d) interest in participating in 15 health-promotion activities within the next month (future). Chi-square analyses were computed for proportion of response differences between perceived health status and current health-promotion behaviors, and between perceived health status and interest in participating in future health-promotion activities. Responses to perceived health status were collapsed into three categories: "excellent," "good" ("very good" and "good" were combined), and "fair." Since only one respondent reported "poor" health status, this person was eliminated from the chi-square analyses. Because 21 different analyses were conducted, the overall ($p \leq 0.05$) level of significance was adjusted to $p \leq 0.002$ (two-tailed) to control for the experiment-wise error rate associated with multiple comparisons. The adjusted p-value was derived by dividing the overall level of significance by the number of comparisons ($0.05/21 = 0.002$) (Munro & Page, 1993).

Sample. Table 1 shows the sample of 53 African-American women's sociodemographic and general health characteristics. The women ranged in age from 20 to 72 years old (M = 47.4, SD = 14.9), had at least a high school education (92%), were employed full-time for wages (63%), reported an annual household income of at least \$35,000 (51%), owned a place of residence (57%), and lived at the current residence for more than two years (72%). Forty-one percent of the women were married/partnered, and 16 women (36%) reported they had children under 18 years old living with them.

The women were on average 64.7 inches (SD = 2.8) in height and weighed an average of 158.4 pounds (SD = 28.1). The women's average body mass index was 26.7 (SD = 4.5), ranging between 19.4 and 38.6. Ranging from 0 to 4, the mean number of reported family history conditions was 1.6 (SD = 1.1), with hypertension (77%) the most frequently reported condition. Out of six choices, the range for personal health conditions was between 0 and 3 (M = 1.0, SD = 1.1), with high cholesterol (43%) the most frequently reported condition.

RESULTS

On a scale of 1 to 5, with 1 representing "excellent" overall health, 98% of the women self-assessed their health status as "fair" or better (M = 2.83, SD = .96), with 75% of them reporting no physical or health impairments that limit activity (see Table 1).

Sixty-seven percent of the women reported that they engaged in physical activity less than three times per week (see Table 2). Of those women, 43% of them engaged in no physical activity. One-third of the women reported that they engaged in physical activity at least three or more times per week. A majority of the women (53%) reported that they ate primarily low-fat foods; however, only 8% of them ate the daily recommended five servings of fruits and vegetables. In terms of tobacco and alcohol use, 85% of the women reported that they do not smoke, 57% of them do not drink, and 42% of them had one to five drinks per week. Over 75% of women reported minimal stress and adequate coping.

A majority of the women (89%) reported interests in participating in at least one of the 15 health-promotion activities within a month (M = 7.1, SD = 4.4). Over 50% of the women were interested in a women's health program, nutrition improvement, health self-care, comprehensive health/fitness evaluation, stress management, weight manage-

TABLE 1. Sociodemographic and General Health Profile (N = 53)

Characteristic	n	%
Marital Status		
Married/partnered	21	41.2
Never married	15	29.4
Divorced/separated	11	21.6
Widowed	4	7.8
Age (years)		
20-25	4	7.5
26-35	11	20.8
36-45	9	17.0
46-55	9	17.0
56-65	15	28.3
>65	5	9.4
Education		
Didn't complete high school	4	7.5
High school graduate	4	7.5
Some college/technical	21	39.6
College graduate	24	45.3
Annual Household Income		
<$10,000	4	8.5
$10,000 – $14,999	2	4.3
$15,000 – $19,999	4	8.5
$20,000 – $24,999	7	14.9
$25,000 – $34,999	6	12.8
$35,000 – $49,999	11	23.4
$50,000 – $74,999	8	17.0
≥$75,000	5	10.6
Employment		
Employed	33	63.5
Retired	12	23.1
Unemployed	7	13.5
Perceived Health Status		
Excellent	5	9.6
Very good	13	25.0
Good	21	40.4
Fair	12	23.1
Poor	1	1.9
Personal Health		
High cholesterol	23	43.4
Hypertension	15	28.3
Diabetes mellitus	6	11.3
Cancer	4	7.8
Cardiovascular disease	4	7.7
Stroke	1	1.9
Family Health History		
Hypertension	39	76.5
Diabetes mellitus	20	39.2
Heart surgery before age 55 years	12	23.5
Cancer	12	23.5

Note: Because of omitted responses, some totals do not sum to *n* = 53. Percentages are adjusted for missing cases.

TABLE 2. Present Health Promotion Behaviors (N = 53)

Behavior	n	%
Physical Activity		
None	22	43.1
Once per week	6	11.8
Twice per week	6	11.8
3 or more times per week	17	33.3
Dietary Fat		
Eat mostly high fat foods	5	9.8
Eat both about the same	19	37.3
Eat primarily low fat foods	27	52.9
Fruits and Vegetables		
1 to 2 servings per day	32	62.7
3 to 4 servings per day	15	29.4
5 or more servings per day	4	7.8
Alcohol Intake		
No drinks per week	30	56.6
1 to 5 drinks per week	22	41.5
6 to 10 drinks per week	1	1.9
Tobacco Use		
Never smoked	27	50.9
Quit smoking	18	34.0
Smokes	8	15.1
Stress/Coping		
Sometimes stressed, coping fairly well	40	78.4
Often stressed, trouble coping at times	11	21.6

Note. Because of omitted responses, some totals do not sum to n = 53 cases. Percentages are adjusted for missing cases.

ment, walking, cancer risk reduction, and aerobics with music (see Table 3). Less than half of the women were interested in cholesterol reduction, heart risk reduction, blood pressure control, alcohol/drug reduction, smoking cessation, and jogging.

There were no statistically significant differences among the women's responses between perceived health status and current health-promotion behaviors, and between perceived health status and interest in participating in future health-promotion activities.

DISCUSSION

Consistent with national data, most of this study's sample of middle-aged African-American women had a family history of hypertension, diabetes mellitus, and cardiovascular disease (U.S. Depart-

TABLE 3. Future Participation in Health Promotion Activities (N = 53)

Activity	n	%
Women's health program	41	80.4
Nutrition improvement	38	77.6
Health self-care	35	71.4
Comprehensive health/fitness evaluation	35	68.6
Stress management	31	63.3
Weight management	30	58.8
Walking	28	54.9
Cancer risk reduction	27	55.1
Aerobics with music	25	50.0
Cholesterol reduction	23	48.9
Heart risk reduction	22	45.8
Blood pressure control	16	34.0
Alcohol/drug reduction	11	22.4
Jogging	8	16.3
Quit smoking	6	20.7

Note. Future was defined as the individual intends to take action within a month. Percentages are adjusted for missing cases and multiple responses.

ment of Health and Human Services, 1998). High cholesterol, hypertension, and diabetes mellitus were the most frequently reported personal health conditions for these mostly healthy, but moderately overweight women. In general, the women were unmarried, well-educated, coping fairly well with stress, reported no physical or health impairments that limit activity, stable in terms of living arrangements, and seemed to have adequate economic resources.

Similar to other study findings, the women reported that they do not engage in regular physical activity, and over one-third of the women reported that they do not engage in any physical activity (Ahijevych & Bernhard, 1994; Felton et al., 1997; McCleary-Jones, 1996). It is imperative that increasing regular physical activity be an area for improvement among African-American women, since findings from other studies revealed that physical inactivity was responsible for about one-third of deaths resulting from coronary artery disease, diabetes mellitus, and certain cancers (McGinnis & Foege, 1993; Powell & Blair, 1994). A majority of women reported that they ate primarily low-fat foods; however, less than 8% of them ate the daily recommended five servings of fruits and vegetables, which are believed to contain substances that are protective against certain cancers (Franceschi et al., 1998; Steinmetz & Potter, 1996). Among this sample of African-American women, there were positive lifestyle behaviors for alcohol and tobacco use. Over 80% of the women reported that they do not smoke cigarettes or drink alcohol in excess.

The women's interests in future, defined as within a month, participation in health-promotion activities were positive and consisted mainly of activities such as women's health, nutrition improvement, comprehensive fitness, stress management, weight management, cancer risk reduction, and moderate physical activity, such as walking. These findings are consistent with other findings in the literature (Martin & Panicucci, 1996; Walcott-McQuigg, Logan, & Smith, 1994). The women in this study did not have an overwhelming desire to engage in vigorous physical activity, such as jogging. This finding should not be viewed negatively because most of the women were interested in moderately intense physical activity, such as walking. Blair and Connelly (1996) found that even a modest amount of physical activity could provide protective health benefits. Less than half of the women were interested in cholesterol reduction, heart risk reduction, blood pressure control, alcohol/drug reduction, and smoking cessation. Over 25% of the women reported a personal health history of high cholesterol and hypertension, and a majority of the women reported they do not smoke or drink. Perhaps, they were currently engaged in other health-promotion activities that were not assessed in this study but that minimized their risks for cardiovascular disease, high blood pressure, and high cholesterol.

There were no statistical differences among the women's responses between perceived health status and current health-promotion behaviors, and between perceived health status and interests in participating in future health-promotion activities. This finding could be related to the fact that perceived health status was fairly high for this group, and, therefore, might not have allowed for detection of an association between perceived health status and present and future health-promotion behaviors. In contrast, one study's findings indicated that perceived health status was associated with preventive health behaviors in Caucasians (Zindler-Wernet & Weiss, 1987).

This study is limited by the convenience sample of mostly educated, middle-aged, middle-income African-American women, whose responses may not represent the larger population of African-American women. Because the sample size was small, we were limited in our control of potential confounders in the analyses. One implication of the study's findings was that, regardless of perceived health status, this particular sample of African-American women had interest in participating in health-promotion interventions in the near future, indicating a preparatory level of readiness for change. These results indicate potential opportunities to engage some African-American women in healthier lifestyle behaviors. There is a need to design health-promotion interventions that address and actively engage various groups of women in their overall health and that match their willingness and readiness to adopt healthier lifestyle behaviors. According to the National Leadership Conference on Physical Activity and Women's Health, women of certain groupings may benefit from particular focus, and perhaps the most effective health-promotion interventions are those that take place at the community level (Jacob's Institute of Women's Health, 1998). To help an individual make a future change, such as to change one's health-promotion practices, health-promotion interventionists must understand the individual's present behavior in the context of that individual's culture.

NOTE

This study was funded by grants provided by the University of California, San Francisco Academic Senate Committees on Research and Equal Opportunity.

REFERENCES

Ahijevych, K., & Bernhard, L. (1994). Health-promoting behaviors of African American women. *Nursing Research, 43*, 86-89.

Ajzen, I. (1985). From intentions to actions: A theory of planned behavior. In J. Kuhl & J. Beckman (Eds.), *Action-control: From cognition to behavior* (pp. 11-39). Heidelberg, Germany: Springer.

American Heart Association. (1999). *2000 heart and stroke statistical update*. Dallas: American Heart Association.

Blair, S.N., & Connelly, J.C. (1996). How much physical activity should we do? The case for moderate amounts and intensities of physical activity. *Research Quarterly for Exercise and Sport, 67*, 193-205.

Blumenthal, D.S., Sung, J., Coates, R., Williams, J., & Liff, J. (1995). Mounting research addressing issues of race/ethnicity in health care: Recruitment and retention of subjects for a longitudinal cancer prevention study in an inner-city black community. *HSR: Health Services Research, 30*(1), 197-205.

Bowlin, S.J., Morrill, B.D., Nafziger, A.N., Jenkins, P.L., Lewis, C., & Pearson, T.A. (1993). Validity of cardiovascular disease risk factors assessed by telephone survey: The Behavioral Risk Factor Survey. *Journal of Clinical Epidemiology, 46*, 561-571.

Bowlin, S.J., Morrill, B.D., Nafziger, A.N., Lewis, C., & Pearson, T.A. (1996). Reliability and changes in validity of self-reported cardiovascular disease risk factors using dual response: The behavioral risk factor survey. *Journal of Clinical Epidemiology, 49*, 511-517.

Brownson, R.C., Jackson-Thompson, J., Wilkerson, J.C., & Kiani, F. (1994). Reliability of information on chronic disease risk factors collected in the Missouri Behavioral Risk Factor Surveillance System. *Epidemiology, 5*, 545-549.

Calnan, M., & Johnson, B. (1985). Health, health risks and inequalities: An exploratory study of women's perceptions. *Sociology of Health and Illness, 7*, 55-75.

Eliason, M.J. (1999). Nursing's role in racism and African American women's health. *Health Care for Women International, 20*, 209-219.

Felton, G.M., Parsons, M.A., Misener, T.R., & Oldaker, S. (1997). Health-promoting behaviors of black and white college women. *Western Journal of Nursing Research, 19*, 654-666.

Franceschi, S., Parpinel, M., La Vecchia, C., Favero, A., Talamini, R., & Negri, E. (1998). Role of different types of vegetables and fruit in the prevention of cancer of the colon, rectum, and breast. *Epidemiology, 9*, 338-341.

Gary, F., Campbell, D., & Serlin, C. (1996). African American women. Disparities in health care. *Journal of the Florida Medical Association, 83*, 489-493.

Giles, W.H., Croft, J.B., Keenan, N.L., Lane, M.J., & Wheeler, F.C. (1995). The validity of self-reported hypertension and correlates of hypertension awareness among blacks and whites within the stroke belt. *American Journal of Preventive Medicine, 11*, 163-169.

Jacob's Institute of Women's Health. (1998). National leadership conference on physical activity and women's health. *Women's Health Issues, 8*, 69-97.

Krieger, N., Rowley, D.L., Herman, A.A., Avery, B., & Phillips, M.T. (1993). Racism, sexism, and social class: Implications for studies of health disease and well-being. *American Journal of Preventive Medicine, 9*, 82-122.

Landrine, H., & Klonoff, E.A. (1997). Conclusions: The future of research on black women's health. *Womens Health, 3*, 367-381.

Martin, J.C., & Panicucci, C.L. (1996). Health-related practices and priorities: The health behaviors and beliefs of community-living black older women. *Journal of Gerontological Nursing, 22*, 41-48.

McCleary-Jones, V. (1996). Health promotion practices of smoking and non-smoking black women. *Association of Black Nursing Faculty Journal, 7*, 7-10.

McGinnis, J.M., & Foege, W.H. (1993). Actual causes of death in the United States. *JAMA, 270*, 2207-2212.

Munro, B.H., & Page, E.B. (1993). *Statistical methods for health care research* (2nd ed.). Philadelphia: Lippincott.

Nickens, H.W. (1995). The role of race/ethnicity and social class in minority health status. *Health Services Research, 30*, 151-162.

Palank, C.L. (1991). Determinants of health-promotive behavior. A review of current research. *Nursing Clinics of North America, 26*, 815-832.

Pinn, V.W. (1996). The status of women's health research: Where are African American women? *Journal of National Black Nurses Association, 8*, 8-19.

Powell, K.E., & Blair, S.N. (1994). The public health burdens of sedentary living habits: Theoretical but realistic estimates. *Medicine and Science in Sports and Exercise, 26*, 851-856.

Prochaska, J.O., & Velicer, W.F. (1997). The transtheoretical model of health behavior change. *American Journal of Health Promotion, 12*, 38-48.

Rosenberg, L., Adams-Campbell, L., & Palmer, J.R. (1995). The Black Women's Health Study: A follow-up study for causes and preventions of illness. *Journal of the American Medical Women's Association, 50*, 56-58.

Sanders-Phillips, K. (1996). Correlates of health promotion behaviors in low-income black women and Latinas. *American Journal of Preventive Medicine, 12*, 450-458.

Siegel, P.S., Frazier, E.L., Mariolis, P., Brackbill, R.M., & Smith, C. (1993). Behavioral Risk Factor Surveillance, 1991: Monitoring progress toward the nation's year 2000 health objectives. *MMWR CDC Surveillance Summaries, 42*, 1-21.

Stein, A.D., Lederman, R.I., & Shea, S. (1993). The Behavioral Risk Factor Surveillance System questionnaire: Its reliability in a statewide sample. *American Journal of Public Health, 83*, 1768-1772.

Stein, A.D., Lederman, R.I., & Shea, S. (1996). Reproducibility of the women's module of the Behavioral Risk Factor Surveillance System questionnaire. *Annals of Epidemiology, 6*, 47-52.

Steinmetz, K.A., & Potter, J.D. (1996). Vegetables, fruit, and cancer prevention: A review. *Journal of the American Dietetic Association, 96*, 1027-1039.

U.S. Department of Health and Human Services. (1998). *Healthy people 2000 progress review: Black Americans*. Atlanta, GA: Centers for Disease Control and Prevention.

Walcott-McQuigg, J.A., Logan, B., & Smith, E. (1994). Preventive health practices of African American women. *Journal of National Black Nurses Association, 7*, 49-59.

Winkleby, M.A., Feldman, H.A., & Murray, D.M. (1997). Joint analysis of three U.S. community intervention trials for reduction of cardiovascular disease risk. *Journal of Clinical Epidemiology, 50*, 645-658.

Zindler-Wernet, P., & Weiss, S.J. (1987). Health locus of control and preventive health behavior. *Western Journal of Nursing Research, 9*, 160-179.

American-Indian Women and Health

Sally J. Stevens

University of Arizona

SUMMARY. Little research has been conducted on the health status and health-related issues of urban American-Indian women, particularly those who are involved with alcohol or drugs (AOD). Given this gap in knowledge, this study assessed the health status along with health care needs and service provision of AOD-involved American-Indian women living in the southwestern United States. Results indicated high levels of AOD use; experiences of sexual misbehavior; multiple pregnancies with adverse outcomes, including stillbirth and loss of child custody; and need for additional health care services. Recommendations include enhancing the education of health care providers with regard to American-Indian women's AOD use and the need for comprehensive, culturally competent, gender-specific AOD treatment services. *[Article copies available for a fee from The Haworth Document Delivery Service: 1-800-342-9678. E-mail address: <getinfo@haworthpressinc.com> Website: <http://www.HaworthPress.com> © 2001 by The Haworth Press, Inc. All rights reserved.]*

KEYWORDS. American Indian, women, health care needs, drug abuse, alcohol abuse

INTRODUCTION

Little research has been conducted on health-related issues of urban American Indians, and even less has been done as it specifically re-

Sally J. Stevens, PhD, is Research Associate Professor, Southwest Institute for Research on Women, University of Arizona, 3912 S. 6th Ave., Tucson, AZ 85714.

[Haworth co-indexing entry note]: "American-Indian Women and Health." Stevens, Sally J. Co-published simultaneously in *Journal of Prevention & Intervention in the Community* (The Haworth Press, Inc.) Vol. 22, No. 2, 2001, pp. 97-109; and: *Prevention Issues for Women's Health in the New Millennium* (ed: Wendee M. Wechsberg) The Haworth Press, Inc., 2001, pp. 97-109. Single or multiple copies of this article are available for a fee from The Haworth Document Delivery Service [1-800-342-9678, 9:00 a.m. - 5:00 p.m. (EST). E-mail address: getinfo@haworthpressinc.com].

© 2001 by The Haworth Press, Inc. All rights reserved.

lates to American-Indian women. Much of the research has focused on alcohol abuse among American Indians, linking it to domestic violence (Norton & Manson, 1995), violent crime (Substance Abuse Letter, 1999), and sexual risk-taking behavior leading to the transmission of HIV and other sexually transmitted diseases (STDs) (Baldwin, Maxwell, Fenaughty, Trotter, & Stevens, 2000; O'Hara, Parris, Fichtner, & Oster, 1998). Other research has indicated that the use of alcohol and other drugs (AOD) is related to morbidity and mortality, especially in relationship to accidents, suicide, and homicide (Baldwin et al., 2000). While death rates linked to alcohol use are still higher for American-Indian men (26.5%) compared to women (13%), the overall rate is 5.6 times that of the overall U.S. rate. Except for Haitians, American Indians have the lowest life expectancy of any population in the Northern Hemisphere (Winik, 1999).

Alcohol and drug-use treatment providers serving American-Indian women have identified physical, sexual, and emotional abuse as the most frequently mentioned childhood life experiences reported by their clients. For adult experiences, the most frequent life experience was single parenting, followed by physical, sexual, and emotional abuse (CRHPR, 1995).

American Indians, particularly those living on reservations, have high rates of unemployment and poverty; relatively few adults have completed high school. Data from the National Center for Educational Statistics (1993) show that American Indians have the lowest educational level of any minority group. Stevens, Estrada, and Estrada (2000) found that American Indians living on a reservation are more likely to be unemployed and to have not completed high school than those living in an urban setting near the reservation. The same study showed that, while poverty rates were similar for both urban- and reservation-dwellers, they were still considerably lower than that of other ethnic groups.

Between 1994 and 1996, 4.5% of American-Indian mothers drank alcohol during pregnancy (as reported on birth certificates), which is three times the percentage for mothers in the general population. The percentage increased with age, except for American-Indian mothers in the under-18 age group, who drank more than those in the 18 to 19 age group. The percentage of American-Indian women living in the Southwest who drank during pregnancy was slightly less than that reported by all American-Indian women (DHHS, 1998-1999). The percentage of live births with prenatal care beginning in the first trimester was only 66.5% for American Indians, compared to 81.3% for all U.S. ethnic groups. In the Southwest, prenatal care beginning in the first trimester for American-Indian women was much lower than that of American-Indian women living in the U.S. (DHHS, 1998-1999). The infant mortality rate (under 1 year) was 9.3%, which is 22% higher than that of all other U.S. ethnic groups. In Tucson, the infant mortality rate exceeded the U.S. rate by 50% (DHHS, 1998-1999). The three leading causes of infant death for Tucson were congenital abnormalities (31.8%), sudden infant death syndrome (22.7%), and accidents and adverse effects (13.6%).

Given the lack of information on the status of American-Indian women's health care issues and needs, this study was developed to assess health care needs and service provision of AOD-involved American-Indian women.

METHOD

The National Institute on Drug Abuse (NIDA) funded this study which took place in a medium-sized city in the Southwest in 1997. Participants were recruited through targeted (i.e., street outreach) and snowball (word-of-mouth) sampling strategies. Potential participants were encouraged to enroll in a women-centered health study aimed at reducing HIV drug and sex risk behaviors. Once at the study site, potential participants were asked about their age, their drug use and drug treatment involvement to ensure that they met the study criteria. Entrance criteria to the study included (1) being female, (2) being at least 18 years old, (3) not being enrolled in substance abuse treatment within the past 30 days, and (4) either having injected drugs, used crack cocaine, and/or had sex with an injection drug user within the previous 30 days. Those who met entrance criteria were asked to sign a subject consent form and were given a baseline questionnaire that addressed health-related issues including AOD use, sexual abuse, medical care history, current sexual activity, contraceptive practices, and pregnancy and childbirth. After the baseline assessment was administered, participants engaged in a brief intervention program that addressed not only HIV drug and sexual risks, but numerous co-occurring issues, such as alcohol and drug use, sexual abuse, vaginal health, pregnancy and parenting, relationships, homelessness, and unemployment. Active referrals to social, health, and AOD treatment were provided.

SAMPLE

The sample included American-Indian women who were either injection-drug users (IDUs), crack-cocaine users (CCUs), and/or female sexual partners (FSPs) of injection-drug users. Recent drug use was verified by checking recent track marks (for injection-drug users) and/or positive urinalysis results for either heroin, cocaine, or methamphetamines. Verification of women who reported being FSPs was facilitated by the interventionist, who either knew the woman's status or communicated with others within the woman's social network to verify that status. Between February 1998 and May 2000, 87 American-Indian women were enrolled in the study.

RESULTS

The first question this study addressed concerned the demographic characteristics of the American-Indian women who participated. These included age, education, marital status, housing status, work situation, and earned income. Of the 87 women who entered the study, the average age was 34.8 years. Less than one-quarter (21.8%) were between 18 and 27 years of age, 43.7% were between 28 and 37 years of age, and 34.5% were between 38 and 54 years of age. Over half had less than a high-school education (58.6%), although 14.9% had received their GED, and 26.4% had more than a high-school education. With regard to marital status, 44.8% were single; 23.0% were legally or common-law married; 13.8% were living with their sexual partner; and 18.3% were separated, divorced, or widowed. Almost half (47.0%) considered themselves homeless. The majority were unemployed (76.6%), while only 10.5% worked full time, 4.7% worked part time, and 8.2% reported being on leave from work, a homemaker, in school, or disabled. Respondents reported on their earned income during the previous 30-day period. One-third (67.4%) earned less than $500, 19.8% earned between $500 and $999, and only 12.8% earned more than $999 (Table 1).

TABLE 1. Demographic Information (n = 87)

	%	N
Age (mean = 34.8 years)		
18-27 yrs.	21.8	18
28-37 yrs.	43.7	35
38-55 yrs.	34.5	34
Education		
Less than high school education	58.6	51
GED	14.9	13
More than high school education	26.4	23
Marital Status		
Single (never been married)	44.8	39
Married, common law	23.0	20
Living with sex partner	13.8	12
Separated, divorced, widowed	18.3	16
Consider Self as Homeless (n = 83)	47.0	39
Current Work Situation (n = 86)		
Unemployed, laid off	76.7	66
Work full time	10.5	9
Work part time	4.7	4
On leave, homemaker, in school, disabled	8.2	7
Earned Income Past 30 Days (n = 86)		
Less than $500	67.4	58
$500 to $999	19.8	17
More than $999	12.8	11

Almost all of the women used either alcohol, drugs, or both during the 30 days prior to entering the study. All of the women reported using alcohol sometime during their life. Approximately three-quarters (74.2%) used alcohol during the 30 days prior to the interview. Of those who used alcohol in that 30-day period, 66.1% had, on average, consumed more than five drinks per sitting. In addition, past 30-day data indicated that 18.4% were IDUs, 23.0% were CCUs, 6.9% were FSPs, 13.8% were IDUs and CCUs, 14.9% were IDUs and FSPs, 4.6% were CCUs and FSPs, and 16.1% were IDUs, CCUs, and FSPs (Table 2).

Sexual history data are presented in Table 3. The average age of first sexual intercourse was 14.7 years. Sixteen percent reported having first sex when they were less than 13 years of age, 20.6% at 13 and 14 years of age, 37.9% at 15 and 16 years of age, and 25.4% at more than 16 years of age. Close to one-third (28.7%) reported that their first sexual experience was forced, and 32.2% reported that they were

TABLE 2. Alcohol and Drug Use (n = 87)

	%	N
Alcohol Use		
Ever used	100.0	87
Used in past 30 days	72.4	63
If used in past 30 days, had more		
than 5 drinks per sitting (n = 62)	66.1	41
Entrance Criteria		
IDU	18.4	16
CCU	23.0	20
FSP	6.9	6
IDU/CCU	13.8	12
IDU/FSP	14.9	13
CCU/FSP	4.6	4
IDU/CCU/FSP	16.1	14

sexually assaulted by having their private parts touched against their will prior to the age of 13 years. Data on the experiences of sexual assault and rape after the age of 13 years indicated that 31.1% were sexually assaulted or raped by a stranger and 20.7% were forced to have sex with their sexual partner. The average number of sexual partners during the 30 days prior to the interview was 2.1, with the majority (64.4%) reporting one partner.

The average number of pregnancies was 3.9%, with the plurality (19.5%) being those who had five or more pregnancies. Four percent were pregnant, and 3.5% were trying to get pregnant at the time of the interview. Almost one-quarter (24.3%) of the women reported having a stillbirth, and 12.3% reported having more than one stillbirth in their lifetime. Of the women sampled, 10.8% reported having an abortion, and 2.7% reported having more than one abortion in their lifetime. Finally, when the women were asked whether any other children (up to the first six children) were currently living with them, the vast majority reported not having physical custody of these children. Only 20% of the women reported their first-born child to be living with them; 22.8% reported their second-born, 20.4% reported their third-born, 18.8% reported their fourth-born, 10.5% reported their fifth-born, and 16.7% reported their sixth-born to be living with them at the time of the interview.

With regard to contraceptive practices, 77% reported having used some type of birth control sometime during their lifetime. Of those who reported ever using birth control, 70% used pills, 24.3% an IUD,

TABLE 3. Sex History (n = 87)

	%	N
Age of first sexual intercourse (mean = 14.66)		
Less than 13 yrs	16.1	14
13 to 14 yrs	20.6	18
15 to 16 yrs	37.9	33
More than 16 yrs	25.2	22
Forced first sexual intercourse	28.7	25
Sex assault under 13 yrs (touch private parts against will)	32.2	28
Sexually assaulted or raped by stranger (13 years and older)	31.1	27
Forced to have sex with a sex partner (13 years and older)	20.7	18
Number of sex partners past 30 days (mean = 2.13)		
0	20.7	18
1	64.4	56
2 or more	14.9	13
Number of times pregnant (n = 85) (mean = 3.85)		
0	8.2	7
1	10.6	9
2	10.6	9
3	17.6	15
4	15.3	13
5	17.6	15
More than 5	19.5	17
Currently pregnant (n = 73)	4.1	3
Trying to get pregnant (n = 85)	3.5	3
Number of stillbirths (n = 74)		
0	63.5	47
1	24.3	18
More than 1	2.7	9
Number of abortions (n = 74)		
0	86.5	64
1	10.8	8
More than 1	2.7	2
Women's physical custody of their children (for first 6 children) (n = 87)		
Child 1	20.0	13
Child 2	22.8	13
Child 3	20.4	10
Child 4	18.8	6
Child 5	10.5	2
Child 6	16.7	2

5.7% a diaphragm, 37.1% male condoms, 2.9% female condoms, 4.3% spermicides, 20.0% Norplant/Depo Provera, and 5.7% withdrawal. Of those who reported "ever use" of these methods, few reported using these methods during the 30 days prior to the interview. Of the 24.3% who reported ever having used an IUD, only 12.5% reported use in the last 30 days. Past 30-day use (including both occasional and consistent use) for condom users was 34.6%, whereas past 30-day use for Norplant/Depo Provera was 35.7%. For the 5% who reported ever using withdrawal, 25% used withdrawal in the 30 days prior to the interview. Tubal ligation, hysterectomy, and partner's vasectomy status were also queried. Over one-third (35.6%) reported having had either a tubal ligation or hysterectomy, whereas only 1.2% reported that their partner had had a vasectomy (Table 4).

Sexually transmitted disease data are presented in Table 5. Almost one-quarter (21.8%) reported having had hepatitis B, 14.9% hepatitis C, 14.9% gonorrhea, 6.9% syphilis, 0% genital warts, 16.0% chlamydia, 1.1% genital herpes, 4.6% trichomonas, 42.5% vaginal candidiasis, and 0% HPV. Last treatment for these reported sexually transmitted diseases varied between 1982 and 1996.

With regard to health care services, 78.1% reported having some

TABLE 4. Contraceptive Practices: Ever Used and Past 30-Day Use

	%	N		
Ever Used Any Method				
Yes	77	62		
No	23	20		
Method	Ever		Past 30 Days	
	%	N	%	N
Birth control pills	70.0	49	0	0
IUD	24.3	17	12.5	2
Diaphragm	5.7	4	0	0
Male condom	37.1	26	34.6	9
Female condom	2.9	2	0	2
Spermicides	4.3	3	0	0
Sponge	0	0	0	0
Norplant, Depo Provera	20.0	14	35.7	5
Morning after pill	0	0	0	0
Rhythm method	0	0	0	0
Withdrawal	5.7	4	25.0	1
Tubal ligation/hysterectomy	35.6	31	NA	NA
Vasectomy	1.2	1	NA	NA

NA: Not Asked

TABLE 5. Sexually Transmitted Diseases (n = 87)

Condition	%	N	last treated
Hepatitis B	21.8	19	1989
Hepatitis C	14.9	13	1996
Gonorrhea	14.9	13	1990
Syphilis	6.9	6	1983
Genital warts	0	0	----
Chlamydia	16.0	14	1992
Genital herpes	1.1	1	1983
Trichomonas	4.6	4	1982
Vaginal candidiasis	42.5	37	1992
HPV	0	0	----

TABLE 6. Health Care Services

	%	N
Have health care insurance (n = 87)	78.1	68
Place of last vaginal/pelvic exam (n = 87)		
Private doctor or nurse practitioner's office	17.2	15
Community health center or clinic	55.2	48
Hospital or emergency care	16.1	14
Never received one	4.6	4
Other	6.9	6
Did provider ask about AOD history? (n = 82)		
Yes	52.4	43
No	47.6	39
Did provider offer HIV/AIDS information? (n = 83)		
Yes	41.0	34
No	59.0	49
Did provider offer HIV testing? (n = 83)		
Yes	48.2	40
No	51.8	43
Did provider offer HIV counseling? (n = 82)		
Yes	31.7	26
No	68.3	56

type of health care insurance (Table 6). Most recent pelvic examination was reported to be approximately 3 years prior to the interview. When asked about the place of their last vaginal pelvic examination, the majority (55.2%) reported a community health care center or clinic, while 17.2% reported a private doctor or nurse practitioner's office, 16.1% a hospital or emergency care center, 6.9% other/not specified, and 4.6% never having received a vaginal pelvic examination. Of the women who did receive a vaginal pelvic exam, 47.6% reported that their doctor did not ask about their AOD history, 59.0% did not offer HIV/AIDS information, 51.8% did not offer HIV testing, and 68.3% did not offer HIV counseling.

DISCUSSION

This study included a group of drug-involved urban American-Indian women living in the southwestern United States. As such, caution must be used in making generalizations to the wider group of non-drug-involved American-Indian women. For this group, however, the demographic information indicates that these women live below the poverty level, and most are unemployed and have minimal education to further their employment and earning opportunities. Almost half consider themselves homeless and, despite the fact that approximately 90% have had children, only 23% are married or in a common-law relationship.

The vast majority of the women reported using both alcohol and drugs, with alcohol use being particularly high. In part, this AOD use may be a contributing factor for the high percentage of homelessness, unemployment, stillbirths, lack of child custody, and sexually transmitted diseases.

Self-report of sexual assault and rape both prior to and after age 13 was substantial yet similar to levels reported by other ethnic groups of women who enrolled in HIV prevention street outreach projects (Stevens, Gama, Polk, & Estrada, 1995). However, the number of pregnancies reported by this group of American-Indian women was higher than for other ethnic groups of women (Stevens & Estrada, 1999). American-Indian women reported an average of almost four pregnancies while women of other ethnic backgrounds reported an average of just under three pregnancies. However, cultural issues, religiosity, and prohibited governmental funding all contributed to the relatively low rate of abortions. Data on the sizeable number of stillbirths was particularly alarming. While reasons for stillbirths were not queried, the high levels of AOD use may have contributed. Certainly causal relationships here pose questions for further research. Further investigation is likewise warranted to compare the role of AOD use to the reasons why many American-Indian women do not have custody of their children. Data from this study indicated that many of the children were in the custody of child protective services, which means that the parenting competence of their mothers was in question.

Despite the number of abortions, stillbirths, and live births, the women reported relatively low levels of contraceptive use. These data do *not* reflect consistent use, but rather any use of any contraceptives. From the data, it appears that about three-quarters of the women used contraceptive methods sometime in their lifetime, yet less than one-quarter used any type of contraceptive method during the 30 days prior to the interview. Given that approximately one-third of the women had a tubal ligation or a hysterectomy, many women did not recently need other forms of birth control for pregnancy prevention. However, given that the average number of sex partners in the past 30 days was 2.13 and the relatively high-risk levels of sexually transmitted diseases, condom use should still be recommended. It is also interesting to know that only one woman reported that her partner had a vasectomy. These data indicate that these American-Indian women take the primary responsibility for ending/preventing pregnancy.

For the most part, the percentage of women reporting sexually transmitted diseases was similar to other ethnic groups of women enrolled in HIV prevention street outreach projects. The unexpected low rate of hepatitis C–particularly given that 63.2% reported having injected drugs during the 30 days prior to the interview–may indicate that the women may not have received medical treatment or hepatitis C testing at the local health department. In addition, almost half of the women reported that their medical provider did not ask them about AOD use, and thus perhaps did not recommend testing for hepatitis C. However, it appears from the data that, when medical providers did ask women about their AOD history, they also offered HIV testing, HIV/AIDS information, and HIV/AIDS counseling.

From this study, many recommendations for improving the health care and health status of American-Indian women can be made. First, medical care providers must consider AOD use to be a medical issue that should be addressed during routine examinations. Medical care providers should be trained to look for signs and symptoms of AOD use and for concomitant ways to discuss with their clients the negative health consequences of AOD use and abuse. Community health centers and other places where American-Indian women receive services should have culturally competent, trained substance-abuse counselors on staff to whom the medical provider can refer substance-using women. Programs that meet the needs of women, particularly young women, must be developed so that substance use and numerous pregnancies–many of which result in AOD exposed infants, stillbirths, and loss of child custody–do not continue for decades.

Typically, the American health care system provides for the "least restrictive and least costly treatment environment" first. When this fails, a more intensive treatment approach is recommended (Stevens, Murphy, & McGrath, 1999). As multiple treatment failures occur, the health and well-being of women is further compromised. Meanwhile, more pregnancies occur and more children are removed from the home because of the mother's inability to adequately care for her children. This approach has not worked. To adequately address the health of American-Indian women, we must first pay attention to how Indians view health and well-being. Starting with approaches to health that complement the culture, history, and beliefs of Indian people will enhance the overall health of American-Indian women. As noted by Lowery (1998), a balanced understanding of recovery includes healing and spirit. Healing is communal, and it is through relationships that the meaning of life can be obtained. Participating in traditional ceremonies, gatherings, pow wows, and feasts enhances American-Indian women's understanding of the spiritual. By developing comprehensive, culturally relevant, and gender-appropriate approaches, AOD treatment modalities can be rendered more effective, which improves the overall health status of drug-involved American-Indian women.

REFERENCES

Baldwin, J.A., Maxwell, C.J.C., Fenaughty, A.M., Trotter, R.T., & Stevens, S.J. (2000). Alcohol as a risk factor for HIV transmission among American Indian and Alaska Native drug users. *American Indian and Alaska Native Mental Health Research: A Journal of the National Center, 9*, 1-16.
Center for Reproductive Health Policy Research. (1995). So she may walk in balance: Integrating the impact of historical trauma in the treatment of Native-Amer-

ican Indian women. In J. Adlemen & G.M. Enquidanos (Eds.), *Racism in the lives of women*: *Testimony, theory, and guides to antiracist practice* (pp. 345-364). Binghamton, NY: Harrington Park Press.

Department of Health and Human Services. (1998-1999). *Regional differences in Indian health*, Indian Health Service. Washington, DC: Office of Public Health.

Lowery, C.T. (1998). American Indian perspectives on addiction and recovery. *Health and Social Work, 23*, 127-135.

National Center for Educational Statistics. (1993). *Digest of educational statistics*. Washington, DC: Government Printing Office.

Norton, I.M., & Manson, S.M. (1995). A silent minority: Battered American Indian women. *Journal of Family Violence, 10*, 307-318.

O'Hara, P., Parris, D., Fichtner, R.R., & Oster, R. (1998). Influence of alcohol and drug use on AIDS risk behavior among youth in dropout prevention. *Journal of Drug Education, 28*, 159-168.

Stevens, S.J., Estrada, A.L., & Estrada, B.D. (2000). HIV drug and sex risk behaviors among American Indian and Alaska Native drug users: Gender and site differences. *American Indian and Alaska Native Mental Health Research: A Journal of the National Center, 9*, 33-46.

Stevens, S.J., & Estrada, B.D. (1999). *Substance involved women: Ethnic differences, contraceptive practices and HIV risk behaviors*. Presented at the Society for Menstrual Cycle Research: Cycling Towards the Millennium: Interdisciplinary Research on Women's Health, Tucson, AZ, June 10-12,1999.

Stevens, S.J., Murphy, B.S., & McGrath, R.A. (1999, March). *Meeting the needs of women patients*. Paper presented at the HIV/AIDS Services in Drug Abuse Treatment Settings: Expanding Research and Practice, Washington, DC.

Stevens, S.J., Gama, D., Polk, B., & Estrada, A.L. (1995, June). *Women at risk: Sexual transmission of HIV*. Paper presented at the Satellite Conference on AIDS and Drug Abuse, Scottsdale, AZ.

Substance Abuse Letter. (1999, February 17). *Alcohol-related arrests are double for Indians*. PaceCom, Inc.

Winik, L.W. (1999, July 18). We are our own destiny: There's a new generation with a different attitude. *Parade*.

Index

© 2001 by The Haworth Press, Inc. All rights reserved.

T - #0252 - 101024 - C0 - 212/152/7 [9] - CB - 9780789013828 - Gloss Lamination